Depres:

CW00853971

The already drowning Man

Second Edition

John Swallow

First Edition	July	2010
Second Edition	September	2012
.... *Updated*	February	2013

Published by   Lulu Enterprises Inc.

Raleigh

North Carolina - 27607

USA

www.lulu.com

ISBN   978 -1 - 300 -14591 - 2

I am grateful to Dr. Tim Cantopher, a leading Psychiatrist, who has described this book as **"special"** and **"really helpful"**.

He writes.....

"There are many books available to sufferers from depressive illness, but this one is special.

John Swallow emerged from his own illness by facing it and understanding it. In this book he uses his own experience, expressed in an easy to follow style with a powerful use of metaphor, to explain to sufferers and those who care about them what the experience of depression is at each of its stages and what helps or hinders recovery.

If you or someone you care about suffers from this horrid illness, you will find this book really helpful"

Dr. Tim Cantopher
Consultant Psychiatrist
The Priory Group.

Foreword

Although the title of this book doesn't suggest it, (I explain the title in Chapter 4) everyone who has read and reviewed the First Edition of this book about depression believed it was a very **positive** experience for them. In fact the average mark given to the First Edition of the book by over 300 reviewers was 9.1 out of 10. The lowest mark it ever received was 8 out of 10.

It was published in the USA during July 2010 and has sold **mostly** in the USA. But it has also sold in the UK, Europe, Asia and Australasia. So, I hope its' success to date reassures you about its' significance and encourages you to read on.

Now, when I wrote the First Edition I did so based mostly on my **OWN** experience but influenced heavily by what I learned from other sufferers. This Second Edition includes much more of the feedback, comments and experiences I have received from my reviewers and others including Doctors and Psychiatrists.

So this is no longer just about **ME** – it's about how many other sufferers with depression said they feel. And what non-sufferers have told me too.

I also need to explain why it is written the way it is. When you write about something like "Depression"; where you want it to be of help to people, you **have** to treat it **seriously**. And, much as I would love my book to be a best-selling "enjoyable read", I know that many will find **ANY** book about depression difficult to get through. That is especially true for sufferers who often find it difficult to read anything let alone something that may bring their issues to the surface.

And non-sufferers may question why I refer to "drowning" when they don't want their family, friends or loved ones who do suffer to even think about it. But they need to understand that every one of my reviewers or friends who suffers with depression has admitted that they have had "black thoughts" on more than one occasion.

So, in order to explain to non-sufferers what sufferers think about, I have to cover these things honestly. That means facing up to topics which some may find difficult.

Many sufferers benefit from taking prescribed anti-depressants but whereas many of them feel better, some don't. Everyone who suffers with depression would love for anti-depressants to "cure" depression but current drugs only seems to "contain" it. As one long term sufferer I know has explained it to me "Anti-depressants only seem to cloud over the issue where I really want something to resolve the problem". Sadly, it seems that we aren't there yet.

In the absence of a "cure", one of the main reasons for me writing this book was to create a learning environment for both sufferers and non-sufferers whereby they could talk about the "feelings" in order to get a better mutual understanding of depression and how it affects the sufferer.

A number of Psychiatrists and Doctors I have come to know have explained to me that, although anti-depressants are certainly helpful in many cases, the biggest impact can come from family and friends whose support can be **CRITICAL** to the recovery of a sufferer whether or not they are on medication. Those sufferers that don't enjoy that level of support from family and friends can often suffer much more and for longer than they otherwise might.

And the family and friends who do support sufferers can only make a difference if they **"understand"** depression and what their relative or friend who suffers is actually going through.

I have been told that the Mental Health Industry world-wide is significantly underfunded and understaffed. It is therefore often difficult for sufferers to get the medical support and treatment that they need. So, it is even more difficult for family and friends of sufferers, who are critical to the recovery of the sufferer, to get the advice and support to enable them to be effective.

Many sufferers get medication and, if they are fortunate, maybe an hour or so of Counselling each month. But they often spend many more hours each week in the company of family and friends. So, any help given to the family and friends of sufferers can have a **HUGE** "multiplier effect".

Perhaps the biggest difference that could be made to this world-wide problem with depression is where the family and friends closest to the sufferer can be helped to understand depression and how they can be of help. And, in the absence of easy access to the professionals, they can only do that by reading books and articles that are helpful and talking to people who understand depression.

One of the biggest problems seems to be that very little has been written **specifically** to help the family and friends of sufferers understand depression and thereby enable them to be **effective** in helping their relative or friend who suffers.

Of the many reviews I received about the First Edition perhaps the most relevant here is this one from the daughter of a sufferer who wrote:-

"There is so much ignorance in the world about depression. Everyone knows someone with depression, so everyone should read this book and it would help".

So, given the gratifying feedback I received from those who reviewed the First Edition, I wrote the Second Edition of my book based on my original experience but placing more emphasis on the many others I have since spoken with **"to help make a difference"** by enabling as many people as possible to read it.

If I could encourage people to understand depression by reading about how it feels and to talk about it, whether they were a sufferer or family member or friend, then over time the lives of thousands (if not millions) of people might improve? If it worked for me then why not tell other people so it can work for them? Talking about depression is perhaps the most powerful aid to recovery and why many sufferers are referred to Counsellors.

As part of that "philosophy", periodically a few fellow sufferers and I (both men and women who have all read my book and some of whom I have known for 15 years or more) meet up purely for the purpose of sharing some of our "depression stories". We don't talk at a medically qualified level as none of us are qualified to. But most family and friends of sufferers aren't medically qualified either.

Now, everyone who knows me also knows that these "meets" are not "depressing events". Quite often we end up telling some "spiritually uplifting stories and jokes" and generally having some fun.

On one recent occasion, where we all agreed to meet to cheer up one of our friends who has been really ill for years, once he had talked about his issues we shared some stories and jokes. We all ended up laughing so much it really hurt. When we left he hugged me and said "John, that was one of the best nights of my life".

So, the lesson here is that family and friends really do have an important role to play in helping anyone suffering with depression. But, as part of that support, it is important to understand how the sufferer feels and that the sufferer has to want to be there.

Equally, you can't just leave the sufferer with others to deal with their issues unless they are professionals or family and friends who really understand.

One of the sufferers with depression whom I have come to know is a retired lady teacher whose hobby is reading and whom I shall call "Jane". She claims to have read well over 50 books on depression during the last 20 years and tells me that most of them were "dreadful, depressing and unhelpful".

Jane told me that for years she had wanted to find a book to read on depression that would help sufferers like her understand how they feel, or be of help to their family and friends in understanding how a sufferer feels. Until she had met me and read mine she said that she had never found one.

She said that when she read the First Edition of this book she suddenly felt "inspired" and incredibly "relieved". For the first time she was able to explain to friends and family how she felt and, when they read the book, they told her that they understood. Her life was changed. Jane said it was the only book she had read which explained in simple terms the experience and way to self-analyse how a sufferer feels from a sufferers' point of view in such a way that almost anyone could understand it.

But my book is not a "qualified medical book" because I have no medical competence. There are many books written by Doctors and Psychiatrists that claim to explain depression but almost all of them are difficult to read. But there is one that stands out and is definitely worth reading.

If you want to read a **good book on depression** written by a **medically qualified expert** then Jane and I both agree (as do all of the people we have recommended it to) that **the best medically qualified book** we have all read on depression is called "Depressive illness: The curse of the strong" Third Edition by Dr. Tim Cantopher (ISBN 978-1-84709-235-9).

Dr. Cantopher is a Consultant Psychiatrist with the national Private Mental Health-care Professionals - The Priory Group. I have heard him speak on the radio and, unlike most other specialists I have listened to, he has the ability to speak very clearly and make the complex subject of depression much easier to understand.

He was among the 15 Doctors and Psychiatrists who read and re-viewed the pre-publication drafts and First Edition of my book. All of them were so kind to have rated my book as at least "good" with one Doctor describing it as "Excellent - a very useful book which, because it breaks down the sufferers experience into bite sized everyday things that everyone can talk about, it supports communication and helps fill a significant void in useful information available to and specifically aimed at the family and friends of sufferers".

A number of the Psychiatrists and General Practitioners also told me that they have used my book with their patients. One of them is Dr. Tim

Cantopher (mentioned above) who was most kind in describing my book as **"a really valuable contribution to the understanding of the experience of major depression".**

He also very kindly offered to write a piece about the book which is now shown on the first page of the Second Edition and on the back cover. Another was Dr. Mark Porter, General Practitioner who also appears occasionally on BBC television and radio, and is an award winning writer on medical issues for "The Times" newspaper in the U.K.

One of the other Doctors who originally helped me with the First Edition of the book told me then that he felt my analysis which separated people into the two groups of "sufferers" and "non-sufferers" was too rigid. He said that with treatments sufferers can move between the two groups.

I understand what he is saying but, from a sufferers' point of view, the difference is very clear – when you are depressed you know you definitely are not in the group called "non-sufferers". And because anti-depressants or other interventions may take time, sometimes weeks, to begin to help with the symptoms many sufferers are **desperate** to find a **faster** way to improve their feelings when they need to.

So, all of the sufferers I have discussed this with agree with the way I differentiate between the two groups because they are very different and sufferers have no choice about which group they are in at any time and have no easy or "fast track route" between them which enables them to suddenly feel better.

When you are depressed you can only see a world with the two groups. There are many days when a sufferer can feel great so they could easily allow themselves to think they are "cured" and that they are in the group that isn't depressed. But, I prefer instead to always consider myself as an ongoing sufferer who is "enjoying a **really** good day" and I make good use of it. If you work hard at it then most days can be good days. Thankfully, now that I feel I understand depression better and use the Dimensions and Self Analysis to work around it, I find that most days are good days for me.

But, perhaps the most important thing I have learned from everyone who kindly read and reviewed the drafts and First Edition of this book, whether they were Doctors or not, is that what I have written isn't just an abstract idea which has no meaning or relevance to anyone else but me. It seems to have struck a chord in the minds of others, both men and women; some who suffer with depression and others that don't.

And most importantly it seems to have achieved two things:-

- Provided both of the above groups (sufferers and non-sufferers) with a means to talk about it together whereby they can get a mutual understanding of what the feeling is like and how they can both cope with it.

- Provided them both with the basis of a method to analyse and measure it so they can distinguish between, and deal differently with, good days and bad days.

I must also explain that while the book makes references to "man" and "men" it is also aimed at women too. Over half of the sufferers whom I know and have discussed this book with are women and, according to them, they especially relate to what I am saying. So, wherever I refer to "men" please also accept that it also refers to "women".

Equally, I have been told by some women that this book could be of particular help to men they know because it seems to them that men are much less willing to seek medical help and the "self-analysis" approach used in this book might enable men to do the same thing for themselves as a first step towards persuading them to see their Doctor. I've been told of several cases where this has happened.

This book also makes no claim to be an "authoritative Self-Help Guide" for other sufferers. However, I have written it in such a way that it can be and has been used as a practical guide by those who feel it helps them. If by considering the way I self-analyse my feelings it can help others to do the same thing for themselves then maybe it can be of use.

Important disclaimer – Everyone is different and while other sufferers may find some similarities between how they and I feel, it is important that they work with their Doctor, Psychiatrist or Professional Counsellor who is qualified to diagnose and treat their unique condition. I am not a qualified person and this book does not seek to replace or interfere with expert opinion.

So, even though I have had the endorsement of many other sufferers, several Doctors and Psychiatrists, the feelings, observations and ideas expressed by me are mostly my own but influenced heavily by what I have learned in the last 2 years and feedback from other sufferers. I hope that other sufferers can use this book and the analogies within it to continue to help themselves as a way to open up, discuss and explore with others how they feel compared to me.

I have launched a blog site which I will update from time to time about the Second Edition of the book. This replaces earlier websites I launched in 2010.

If you want to follow future developments please refer periodically to it:-

www.thealreadydrowningman.org

INDEX

Chapter

APPENDICES

KEY

Serious feelings	R	Red
Feelings which can most affect the Red feelings	A	Amber (Yellow)
Other feelings which can affect Red and Amber (Yellow) feelings	G	Green

1 - Introduction

I must begin this Introduction with a Statement.

I didn't write this book as a result of intellectual or scientific research or in collaboration with anyone who is a qualified practitioner in any branch of Mental Health. Following my diagnosis about 5 years ago I was asked by a Counsellor to write down my feelings and what started as a few pages of notes very soon became 30 pages and the basis of the First Edition of this book.

What started as a personal exercise by me and written by me was only ever intended to help **ME**. Only when I asked some close friends to look at it and see if it made any sense did it begin to snowball when they and more people they knew asked if they could read copies of the first draft.

Since then I have been touched and humbled by the hundreds of comments I have received all saying that they either fully understand what I have written or that they feel exactly like me. But, let me be clear, I have absolutely no claim to even the slightest competence in the area of Mental Health.

However, a couple of the "non-medical" books I have read on the subject of depression and which have helped me weren't written by practitioners either. I have tried to read some of the text books but they were typically written by experts for other specialists in their Profession. They certainly weren't aimed at someone like me who has no expertise in their "field" and I have inevitably got lost in the technical detail which supports their science. In fact, the more I read their text books then the worse my understanding seemed to get.

So this book is written by me in a very simple style to explain my experience with and analysis of depression and what I have learned from my discussions with other sufferers and non-sufferers with no links to accepted technical expertise. If others can relate to what I have written then that is good; not least because it means what I have written is relevant to more and more people.

After I was diagnosed by my Doctor as having depression and having analysed the feelings that I can remember experiencing over many years, I came to the conclusion that I have actually been "suffering" with depression not just for 5 years but since I was 9. So, if I am right, that means I appear to have "lived" with "depression" for over 50 years now.

One would assume that there isn't much about it I don't know. The reality is quite the opposite. Until I was diagnosed I had never considered that I might suffer with depression and only now am I really beginning to learn about it. In fact, like many other sufferers I know, I have often said to myself and others, "I never get depressed". I may even have said it when I was depressed without ever realising why I felt like I did at the time. Many other sufferers have told me that they know they have done **exactly** the same thing.

Another thing I should mention here is that there are a number of different types of depression in addition to mine and I'm not qualified to differentiate between them. When I wrote the First Edition of this book I wasn't sure if my analogies might work for sufferers with other types of depression. In the event, I have found that almost all of the sufferers I have spoken with agree with me and way I have described how I feel.

So, given the random nature and numbers of people I have spoken with, I feel reassured that what I have written must apply statistically to a range of different types of depression.

But, why did I feel "qualified" to write a book about it?

Good point! I am not "qualified" in a technical sense, but I did share the first drafts with over 150 people (both sufferers and non-sufferers, men and women, friends and many who did not know me personally and 11 Doctors) before the First Edition was published and they all seemed to feel that my "experience and analysis" did qualify me to write about it and it did help all of them to understand a little more about what is widely regarded as a very complex subject. So, both they and I felt it was worth sharing and the subsequent feedback I have had has supported that view.

The fact that sufferers felt it helped them, even if my own experience was sometimes a little different to their own, was important to me. But I felt it was especially important if it helped anyone who is **NOT** a sufferer but has a member of their family, a loved one or a friend who is suffering with depression. They usually want to know how they can be of help, or at least find out something about why their relative or friend is so often "very odd"!

In one of the semi-technical books that I read called "Malignant Sadness – The Anatomy of Depression" by Lewis Wolpert – Third Edition (ISBN 978-0-571-23078-4) there is a part which describes 9 feelings (page 17 of his book) that people suffering with depression might complain about.

According to Lewis Wolpert, and apparently as classified in the Diagnostic and Statistical Manual of Mental Disorders – Fourth Edition (DSM-IV) as published by the American Psychiatric Association, the 9 feelings are as follows:-

- Depressed mood for most of the day
- Diminished interest or pleasure
- Significant gain or loss of weight
- Inability to sleep or sleeping too much
- Reduced control over bodily movements
- Fatigue

- Feelings of worthlessness or guilt
- Inability to think or concentrate
- Thoughts of death or suicide

Now, if consistently over a 2 week period,

- you have 4 of these feelings then you are **mildly** depressed.
- you have 6 it is regarded as a **medium** depression.
- you have 8 or more then it is **severe**.

It is well known that anyone who reads a medical dictionary is likely to end up feeling like they are suffering from everything they read about. But, the feelings in the list did make me think about and start to analyse how I felt on a daily basis and it is true that, from time to time, I did feel all 9 of the "feelings". Hardly ever did I feel them **ALL** of them **at the SAME time.** But I did feel **ALL** of them **at SOME time.**

I have already explained that my book is not based on any scientific research. It is based on an analysis of **MY** feelings and the way I have found to explain to myself and those around me how I feel. And, having discussed more recently with hundreds of other people whom I know suffer with depression, they have all told me that they understand what I am saying.

The difficulty for most sufferers I have spoken with is that they just can't find **ANY** way to accurately describe how they feel in such a way that others would understand; even their own family and friends. Most of them have told me that the approach I have taken is the first time they have begun to understand and analyse depression for themselves and my analysis seems much better than anything that they have previously come up with.

I do not intend to personalise this with loads of specific "real life" examples from my own experience as this book is no longer just about **ME**. But I will explain that most of my career has had to do with either Manufacturing or Computing or Business and I have worked Internationally in Senior Management roles on Multi-million dollar projects with some World renowned companies in those fields. I have enjoyed some great successes in spite of feeling what, at the time, I just described as like being "under the weather".

When I was given the objective by a Counsellor to write down my feelings I began by using my business analysis skills which came naturally to me. I began by thinking about how I might describe to others how I actually felt. I was used to analysing things with numbers so I felt that I needed to find a method that did the same for my feelings. For me, linking **"feelings"** to **"numbers"** is a fascinating concept. Interestingly, as I became more and more motivated to develop this process I found it helped **ME** deal with how I felt. It started to give me a structure within which to live and work with my depression.

Having developed the method included in this book I can now describe how I feel in almost a **"clinical"** way. And, once they have completed the Self Analysis Chart in Appendix 1, so can any other sufferer. It enables me to put numbers to depression in a way that can give me and others a real sense of measure. It has also helped me to focus on the feelings which are most affecting me at any point in time and enabled me to deal with them individually. At any time of day I can work out what my "priority feeling" is.

Without question, the best outcome of what I have learned is being able to understand how I feel in each of the Dimensions (feelings). I will explain the term "Dimensions" shortly in Chapter 2 – The Model. Most of the sufferers I know and who have read this book have said to me that the ability I have given them to identify the "priority feeling" and put a number to it has been of the greatest help to them.

One of the **most important** comments ever made to me was by a long-term sufferer who said:-

"You can't deal with depression all at once. You have to deal with it bit by bit. And this really has helped me to do that"

So, why do I think that I started feeling depressed when I was only 9 years old?

Well, when I was 9, I suffered with Glandular Fever and was off school for about 5 weeks. I've certainly not been told about any known direct link between Glandular Fever and Depression. Maybe the Medical Profession knows of hundreds of links or perhaps there is just one. Or maybe there isn't even one proven link.

But I do know that in my case, prior to the Glandular Fever I was apparently an intelligent, energetic and enthusiastic student (according to family and friends) whereas, after that, everything I did at school required a real mental effort. I can actually remember saying to my parents and Doctor "I'm not sure why but since having Glandular Fever I do feel **very** different mentally. My brain doesn't seem as clear or work as well. It feels foggy and slower and I always feel tired".

It was a few months after this that I was assessed by a leading and world renowned Psychiatrist in London, England who was introduced to us by a family friend (who was also a Doctor), to find out if the Glandular Fever had affected my "intelligence". I recall being given the "all-clear" and was assessed as having a very high I.Q. (Intelligence Quotient).

So, whatever happened when I was 9, it hadn't affected my intelligence but it did seem to have affected my ability to process information in some form. Since then there has always been this "Fog". Sometimes, when I feel depressed, the fog is quite thick. At other times, when I don't feel depressed, there is no fog and I can "reason" and think clearly.

I still achieved success at school and was often top of my class in most subjects but it wasn't anything like as easy to me as it seemed prior to that. Suddenly, to be as good as I was before, I had to work really hard. **Much** harder than before, when everything I did seemed so easy and natural to me.

And, to be honest, nothing seems to have come as easily to me ever since. I have always felt I have had to work hard to achieve the best results. Fortunately, I enjoy hard work and I do achieve. But, quietly, I do wonder now what life would have been like if I still had that feeling of ease with which I found things before I was 9.

Every sufferer I have spoken with agrees with me that trying to find a way to describe depression to someone else is extremely difficult so I began my process of analysis by trying to describe it to myself. Having thought about it for some time, I came up with the image in my mind that whatever was going wrong in my brain felt a little like I was "mentally drowning".

Now, even I thought the idea of "mentally drowning" was quite strange at first. But the more I have got used to it; I have accepted that, for me, the analogy really works and it does help me analyse it and deal with it. And, most importantly, lots of other sufferers I have spoken with seem to like my analogy **and it works for them too.**

To me, the feeling of "mentally drowning" was like the brain was already trying to do far too much, mainly in my subconscious over which I had no control, and anything I wanted my brain to do made it worse and my brain seemed to put what I wanted at the bottom of its' "to do list" and I had to fight really hard to get my brain to do it.

Now it might be that if you are a sufferer you won't easily accept my analogy. Maybe for you it is different. Maybe the "Dimensions" I use don't exactly relate to how you feel. Or that the scale of the measures I use don't fit with your condition. Maybe you have more "Dimensions" or perhaps you have less. They could obviously be different "Dimensions" in terms of how you feel.

I totally accept that if you are a sufferer then your experience may be different because I don't believe any two sufferers are **exactly** the same. But what I have found from discussing it with other sufferers is that depression is **NOT** just **ONE** thing. It isn't just **ONE feeling** but a **very complex MIX of several different feelings**. And, most of the sufferers I have spoken with think that the ones I have chosen are in most cases exactly the same as theirs or at least a good representation of the feelings they have too.

So, other sufferers and I may not all agree on the exact description of how it feels to me, but everyone seems to agree with my analogy that it is **"a very complex MIX of several different feelings"**. And that it is difficult for the sufferer to understand and differentiate between these feelings let alone begin to describe them to others. They accept that my analogy is at least one way of helping those who do not suffer with depression to get a better understanding of what it might be like for their relative or friend who does suffer.

Now, I am told that sufferers find what follows next very easy to understand. For them it is very real!

However, if you **DON'T** suffer with depression, then in order to help you really begin to understand what I mean about my metaphorical analogy with "mentally drowning" I need to ask you to do something. And it will help you if you concentrate and avoid any distractions for the next few moments because I want this to feel very **"REAL"** for **YOU.**

Imagine for a moment that you and some friends are on a ship that is going out to sea for a day. After a while you go for a walk alone around the deck and you lean against a railing which suddenly breaks and you have now fallen off the side of the ship and into the sea. The ship was already miles (kilometres) out of the harbour and the water is obviously deep. Worse still, no-one has noticed you falling off the side of the ship and it just carries on sailing away from you. Even worse than that is the fact that you can't swim properly and you are beginning to sink. You take in a bit of water in your mouth and nose and you are beginning to panic. You start to thrash around increasingly wildly in an attempt to keep yourself afloat.

Now, have you got a picture in your mind and a **real** sense of panic and how it might feel to be alone in the middle of the sea and drowning?

For hour after hour you struggle to stay afloat and although you have taken in and spat out a huge amount of water you still have not drowned. But for every second of your time in the water your mind is concentrating on surviving and how to stay afloat and you are never sure for how much longer you can do it. It's exhausting and by now you are really tired. But, absolutely one hundred percent of your entire brain and body is totally focussed on survival. You can't think about anything else. Even though you are physically exhausted by the effort, how could you possibly think about anything else when you are trying to stay alive?

Now, let's move your imagination back to the "safety of land".

Imagine that your brain is doing this "survival thing" subconsciously every second of every day and at times you are consciously aware of it (when it is bad) but quite often you are not (when it is not so bad). Your brain subconsciously never stops trying to prevent you from "mentally drowning" even though you might be at home and totally safe and lying in bed.

As a sufferer it feels to you as though your brain is malfunctioning and doing its' best (and totally on its' own) to recover from the process or whatever it thinks is going wrong and help find ways around the problem for you. There is nothing **YOU** can do to stop it or make it better or worse. But, at its' worst and as it is happening, you find it difficult to cope with anything else because your brain is subconsciously fully occupied in doing its' "own thing".

So, day by day even though your brain is off doing its' "own thing", you are trying to live a normal life as if nothing like this is happening. Everyone around you from family and friends to colleagues at work are carrying on like everything is normal.

And for them everything **IS** normal.

But for you to respond to them "normally" often requires "super human" effort to appear normal when all the time you don't understand yourself what is happening. Your brain seems to get distracted and interrupted by processes inside it over which you have no control while you are in the middle of doing whatever you want or need your brain to do.

I also need to explain here that, although I have already and will continue to use a number of water based analogies, I don't want you to begin thinking that I mean a sufferer with depression has water rushing around inside their head. **They don't.** This isn't "water on the brain"!

Let me take a moment to share with you how I and many others I know have described how it **actually** feels **physically**.

I understand from the "experts" that the cause of depression is a chemical imbalance within the brain. The degree of imbalance changes at various times of the day and night and anti-depressant drugs are designed to help restore and maintain the balance. But, whatever the cause, when you are depressed your brain **feels** as if it has become physically abnormally **heavy.**

It feels as though something is gently pressing down on your brain and against it from all sides. It is similar to a very bad head cold or, for those of you who have ever drunk a little too much alcohol, a "hang-over" but without the pain. The important point here is that **depression isn't "painful".** Sometimes you wish there was some pain to help you work out how bad it is.

But the consequence to a sufferer is a bit like their brain has stopped behaving normally and things they are thinking about feel as though they are being swirled around and "swept away" out of their reach. The effect is a bit like building a jigsaw where someone is constantly removing pieces the sufferer has already placed and hiding them or moving the other pieces they are still looking for without them knowing.

In order to remember things or how to do things, a sufferers' brain has to work very hard to find and piece all of the bits of the jigsaw back together again. Now, you might expect a sufferers' brain would try to work harder and faster in order to catch up. But, instead of working harder and faster to catch up, a sufferers' brain seems to slow down and give them less and less of its' ability to work for them. They have no choice but to try and ignore it and, to the extent that they can, get on with their life as "normal".

When you are really depressed it is as if your brain is almost stopped. In order to explain it to non-sufferers I have tended to use sea waves which everyone can picture as a vivid way to get them to imagine how distracted and pre-occupied your brain might be if you were in the process of "mentally drowning" but you still had to get on with other things as well.

The biggest problem for most sufferers is that no-one they know personally seems to understand depression or how they feel. And because family and friends or colleagues at work can't see or don't know that you are ill, they have no way of taking it into account. How many times have you heard people suggest to a sufferer who seems depressed that they should just "Snap out of it"! You need to take a moment to try and understand it from the sufferers' point of view.

To try and help you **understand,** let's continue with the theme of drowning.

Imagine in the earlier analogy if someone on the ship had found the broken deck-rail, realised you were missing and that you must have fallen overboard and the ship did turn around to look for you and they did eventually find you several hours later. Can you imagine that the ship is now right beside you?

Now, if instead of imagining what it is like to be "drowning" in the water, what would it feel like if you were one of the people on deck and that you saw your relative or friend "drowning" in the deep water at the side of the ship below you.

How "sensible and logical" would you feel it would be if, in your "desperate" attempt to be of help to your relative or friend who was drowning, the only thing you did was to shout out **"Stop drowning"?**

No attempt by you to get them out of the water. No life belt thrown to them. No boat lowered to go out and get them. Don't you think that the person in the water would love to "Stop drowning" if there was even the remotest possibility of them being able to do so? What do you think they have been trying to do for the last few hours?

So, saying "Snap out of it" to someone with depression is almost certainly the most stupid thing anyone could say.

Someone suffering with depression even has difficulty in doing simple things which they themselves might do easily on another day at another time. But during a depressive moment there is little or nothing they can do. And I do mean here that they **REALLY CAN'T**. It's like a form of mental paralysis.

Another thing to point out here is that most people associate drowning with death and that if you were to drown it would all be over for you in a matter of seconds. To a depressed person that would be sweet relief to their problems if their depression passed away in seconds.

But it doesn't.

In order to understand how bad it can feel to a sufferer let me ask you now to think about the following. Once again, try to make this feel **real** for yourself because I know it does for sufferers. They really identify with this.

Imagine you are in the water and "drowning" but to your surprise after a minute you are still alive.

Imagine how much energy it has taken you to survive for that whole minute. It would be totally exhausting wouldn't it?

So, let's stretch your imagination a bit further. Now try really hard to imagine yourself in this situation.

How would you feel if you hadn't drowned but you were **still** drowning after ....

- 2 minutes?
- 10 minutes?
- 1 Hour?
- 1 Day?
- 1 Week?
- 1 Month
- 1 Year?

Yes, I really mean a year!

Where it never actually ends and you know it is **NEVER** going to end?

Where every day for you is a constant struggle to avoid "drowning". Where in addition to avoiding "drowning" you also try to lead a normal family life? Can you imagine how exhausting that would be?

On a good day a sufferer may only slightly feel like that. On a bad day they can't feel anything else.

So, if you don't suffer with depression and you want to try and understand how it feels, imagine trying to stay "mentally alive" in addition to what you **normally** do every day no matter what the "waves" in your brain are doing to you and no matter how huge they are.

Well that's what depression is like. It's just that it is quietly happening in your head and no-one can see it. And you have to cope with it all of the time and, sometimes, that can seem like a full time "job".

Let me conclude this introduction with a further analogy using the theme of water.

And this is arguably the most important analogy I use in the whole book.

- If you **DON'T** suffer with depression then, in this analogy, you are **ALWAYS** on land or on the ship and you are always "**DRY**".

- If you **DO** suffer from depression then, in this analogy, **you are ALWAYS in the water. You**

NEVER get out of the water and you are always "WET".

So, if you don't suffer with depression but know someone who does then always remember, whatever else you might talk to them about or do while you are together, they are **always** in the "water" and **"WET"** whereas you are always **"DRY"**. As long as you are both in such different situations then you can **NEVER** feel exactly the same.

When a sufferer is well life can be so **very easy** for them because they know just how awful and difficult it is when they are depressed. That is why people with depression sometimes seem extremely happy when they feel well because it feels to them like they have been "set free" for a while.

It is perhaps like the comparison of running up a steep hill and then running back down again. Going up it is difficult and slow and you get very tired. When you are coming down it is difficult to stop yourself from running too fast and you feel exhilarated and great.

The next Chapter 2 is called "The Model" which builds on this analogy of "water" to help explain some of the differences in how a sufferer might feel during depression and to begin the process of analysis.

2 - The Model

Scientists use "Models" (these are like sets of instructions on how to do things) to create a framework or way of doing things such that whenever they carry out an experiment they can recreate the same set of conditions and thereby get a consistent set of results.

In creating a "Model" for you to use for depression I am trying to establish something which is consistent for you (whether you are a sufferer or part of the family or a friend) and those around you. As a sufferer, you may want to change the terminology I use to describe certain feelings you have or you may want to change the scale I use. If you do and it works for you then go ahead. But the structure and method should remain the same.

Let me begin this Chapter by acknowledging an excellent non-technical book about depression written and illustrated by Matthew Johnstone called "I had a Black Dog" (ISBN 978 – 1 84529-589-9). A "Black Dog day" is how Sir Winston Churchill used to describe the days when he suffered with a bad period of depression.

I think Matthews' book is an excellent way to pictorially explain what depression is all about (it is almost entirely made up from clever pictures), especially to children in a family. It is an excellent way to help people around you begin to understand the concept of depression. It's interesting that he too uses water and waves in one of his illustrations to explain "isolation". I had already begun to develop my "water based analogy" long before I bought and read his book but I really felt a strong link to the concept on that page.

As an engineer and business analyst, I am much more used to dealing with facts and figures. I am far less used to dealing with "philosophical or semantic" ideas and concepts. My life has been built around the certainty associated with various forms of scientific analysis and the results.

In engineering they typically deal with numbers and scientific certainties. We know from physics that there are 3 Primary Dimensions (typically described as length, width and height) and arguably the 4th Dimension is time. There are also 3 states of matter; solids, liquids and gases. Each of these has properties which describe and distinguish them and among these are density, temperature and mass. In gases and liquids we can also use pressure.

It really doesn't matter what these names mean or what they describe but it is important for you to understand that each of them has different units of measure which enable us to use numbers to compare one situation with another.

In medicine we are used to Doctors taking our blood pressure and temperature. Because Doctors know from experience what the "norms" are (i.e. what the numbers are for normal blood pressure and temperature) this information enables the Doctor to measure your blood pressure and temperature when you are ill, compare your results with the "norms" and help them work out what might be the reason for the illness. The Doctor can then decide what to do or what medicine to prescribe in order to make you feel better.

Now I know that Medicine is far more complex than that but the numbers for blood pressure and temperature do offer some basic numeric diagnostic measures Doctors can use which give at least some indication of where to start their more detailed diagnosis.

The difficulty with the laymans' perception of Psychiatry and how the brain works is that they do not know of any numbers that are "widely used" to do with measurements of the brain other than I.Q. (Intelligence Quotient). If there are, then no-one told me about them when I originally wrote the book.

Since publishing the Second Edition of this book I have been made aware of The Hamilton Rating Scale for Depression (HRSD) which is described on Wikipedia (www.wikipedia.com). The original version was developed in 1960, contained 17 questions and is known as HRSD-17. Another version which enhanced the process is known as HRSD-29.

Hamilton did not see his Scale as suitable for Diagnosis but the article on Wikipedia does refer to other scales. I am not qualified to comment on them but invite anyone who wants to know more to look them up.

So, when the brain has problems with how it works, how do you or I, a Doctor or a Psychiatrist, work out where to begin? What is a normal brain and what does it "look" like. How does yours or mine compare with the norm?

And when the process by which your brain works goes through a change how do you measure and describe it in more precise terms than "feeling well" or "feeling ill"?

When I began to analyse my idea of "mentally drowning", I was aware that the metaphor for "water" in which I felt I was "mentally drowning" could take many forms. It could be like the sea, a river, or a lake. If you can imagine it, if you were drowning in any one of these then in each case your circumstances might feel strangely different. You might still feel as if you were "drowning" - but in a different way.

For example, a lake might be quite still but it might be very deep and as you "drown" you might just slowly and peacefully sink. A river could be very shallow but fast flowing so you could be swept away violently and at great speed over the rocks. The sea could have mountainous waves which crash down on your head each time you surface as if you were deliberately being pushed under.

Can you see how you might still feel like you are "drowning" but each of the experiences could be very different?

Now, using my engineering skills, I began to "see" some physical and dimensional differences between the feelings I felt. So, I started to apply these different scenarios to the physical Dimensions of **height, length and width** in ways that can describe how some of the feelings of depression can affect you. And I called each of these different scenarios a **"Dimension"**.

As far as the physical nature of the "water based analogy" is concerned then:-

- One feeling is like being pounded by huge waves in the sea – this is comparable to the Dimension of **height** as you rise and fall with each wave.

- The second feeling is a little like being swept away in a fast flowing river – this is comparable to the Dimension of **length** in terms of how far you travel and how fast.

- The third feeling is like being close to or miles (kilometres) away from a shore where you can get help – I compare this to the Dimension of **width;** like the width of a lake or the distance from the shore to the horizon.

In addition to the above 3 feelings (Dimensions) there are the other feelings which I compare to time and temperature or climatic conditions such as the wind and rain, and even the effect of the sun. These will become clearer as you get further into the Dimensions.

So the "Model" I am trying to create for you to visualise and "artificially experience" is one based upon several "Dimensions" each of which represents a different **"feeling"** and explores the way in which you might be affected by this water based metaphor for "mental drowning".

What I find interesting now when I analyse how I feel at any given time is that I can express in numbers how I feel in each of the separate Dimensions. If you are a sufferer then, by the end of the book, you will also be able put numbers to the way you feel too.

I know from talking to the family and friends of sufferers that one of the most difficult things for them to understand is that for any sufferer their depression doesn't always feel the same at different times on the same day **even** for the same person. I would describe depression as a **constantly varying mixture of feelings.** You can feel fine in one Dimension (feeling) but really bad in another. Occasionally you can feel fine in all of them. But for a sufferer during each and every day the mix and intensity of the various feelings will always change.

Often, circumstances in a sufferer's daily life might require them to do something when they are feeling really ill with depression because their family or their job demands it regardless of how they feel at the time. Whatever they have to do in circumstances like that may require "super human" effort compared to other people and, afterwards, for no obvious reason to the others, the sufferer may be so exhausted they have no alternative but to go to bed. In much the same way that saving yourself from drowning can be both mentally and physically exhausting, when a sufferer is depressed it can also be both mentally and physically exhausting.

Another thing to mention here before we move into the next Chapters and the descriptions of the various "Dimensions" (feelings) is that the sensitivity for anyone with depression may vary between the "Dimensions" (feelings) at any time. So on some days a sufferer may hardly be affected by anything that happens whereas on others even the slightest thing can affect them. And, just to make things even more complex, the effect might be only slight in one Dimension but, for absolutely no obvious reason, huge in another.

Over time a sufferer can begin to learn about the sensitivities they feel and they can take some steps to try and help themselves avoid aggravating how they feel at any given time. But, typically, whatever they do only has a very small effect. Where a sufferer knows that certain things adversely affect them then it is important for them to let family and friends around them know what these things are so they can understand how they may be affected and to what extent the family and friends may be able to help.

Apparently, there are well over 200 million people in the World at any given time being treated with anti-depressant drugs (with up to 500 million people actually suffering with depression at any one time) and I know some people who are so ill that they really have no choice but to take anti-depressants to help them cope. My impression is that, unlike some medical conditions for which there is a known "cure" or treatment, depression can only be "controlled" by drugs because there is currently no cure.

If there was a cure then every depressed person could complete their treatment and with confidence come off it. They could "metaphorically" swim to the shore, get out of the water and get **"DRY"**. And I doubt if there is one sufferer in the World who wouldn't just love to do that. Being out of the "water", no longer "mentally drowning" and "dry" is the ultimate ambition.

But in the same way that fish only live in the water and we live on land, people with depression are consigned to this metaphorical "mental limbo land" where they have to co-exist somewhere between wet and dry. Where sufferers live in the wet and deal with people who are only ever dry. And the non-sufferers who are the people in the dry wonder why a sufferer is always **"WET"** and why they don't just "snap out of it", get out of the water and get **"DRY"**. But, sadly, sufferers can't.

As one of the methods to help with the analysis and to differentiate between the different "Dimensions" (feelings) I've used a popular prioritisation technique which is widely used in Project Management.

It is called the "RAG" (Red, Amber, and Green) System; for each feeling just like traffic lights where:-

- Red   is a critically important item that is Urgent
- Amber (Yellow)   is an important item which needs looking at
- Green   is an item that is under control and OK.

The way in which I apply "RAG" in this book is to try and categorise the different feelings as not all of them are as "important" or as intense as the others.

They all do have an effect on each other but while some, typically the Red ones, are difficult to affect positively if at all, the Green ones can be affected and may either directly or indirectly impact positively on the Amber (Yellow) and Red ones.

So, to bullet this point again so that in relation to my analogy it is clear:-

- Red   The most important and serious feelings
- Amber (Yellow)   The next most important feelings which most affect the Red ones

- Green   The other feelings
                          which can also affect
                          the intensity of the Red
                          and Amber (Yellow)
                          ones.

I have summarised this method in the **KEY** after the Index on Page 14.

But, let us also be clear, unlike a "Green issue" as used in Project Management, which defines an item that is "under control and OK", a Green "feeling" is still a problem for the sufferer. It is just less of a problem than the Red or Amber (Yellow) ones.

When you get to the end of the book I have included some Appendices to help with the ongoing support and analysis for the sufferer, their family and friends. Let me begin to describe them here.

Appendix 1 - at the end of the book, sufferers will get the chance to complete the Self Assessment Chart I use for myself and which I know many other sufferers use to help themselves. For the first time, sufferers can assess how they feel and "put a number to it".

Appendix 2 – this is aimed at helping family and friends by giving them a "rough guide" on how to interpret the sufferers' scores.

Appendix 3 - at the end of each Chapter which covers a new "Dimension" (feeling), I end with a quick one paragraph **Summary** of the main points to do with that "Dimension" (feeling). To help you remember them, in Appendix 3 you can find a Quick Reference - Bullet Point Summary for all 10 of them together in one place.

Appendix 4 - I have included a blank form which can be used either as a template or a place where the sufferer can record the things which either help them feel better with each of the feelings I have identified (or their own) and the other things which make them feel worse.

Finally, it is important for family and friends to understand that sufferers will **always** have a score above 10 and may occasionally have a score above 90. They will **never** have a score of zero even on a day when they feel great.

That is because there are 10 Dimensions and I have deliberately given each a minimum score of 1 so the minimum total score you can have is 10. The fact that you will **always** have a score of at least 10 acts as a reminder that you always need to be careful.

The reason for having a minimum score is that I don't believe a sufferer is ever completely "cured" even when they are receiving treatment and feel great. There is always the possibility that they might suddenly feel unwell. And to acknowledge that possibility is an important way to support their treatment and the way they live their life.

Now, let's move on to the next Chapter and the description of the various Dimensions.

3 - Dimension 1 – Sea Wave

Red

- *This refers to the overall feeling of Depression.*

Clearly, if you were **really** drowning, it is a bit academic for anyone to say to you that one feeling of drowning is worse than another. But I am beginning with the one feeling to the sufferer that is most similar to drowning in the sea because of all of the different feelings to do with depression and which I describe as Dimensions, then the "Sea Wave" is the worst and is the basis for, and perhaps the result of, all of the others.

You will notice under the heading at **the top left of this page** I have included the title **"Red"**. This is the place in all 10 of the Dimensions where I classify each of them in terms of how serious this feeling is. As you progress through the book, you will see the level of each Dimension at the beginning of the Chapter. Clearly, Dimension 1 is Red.

Also, under the Chapter number and Dimension name I include a reference to the main feeling(s) referred to in this Dimension. So, as shown above, the "Sea Wave" really covers the overall feeling of **"Depression"**.

The sea can often produce waves which are over 60 feet (20 metres) high. There are occasionally freak waves which are over 100 feet (30 metres) high. Apparently, it has been shown that Tsunamis can produce waves of over 300 feet (100 metres) high. But, if you are drowning, I am sure that waves of as little as 1 foot (30 centimetres) high can be pretty dreadful. I think anything above 5 feet (150 centimetres) high would be way too much for most people when they are struggling to stay afloat.

I believe that the sea provides the best comparison as to the feeling of "mentally drowning" that underpins anything else a sufferer might feel. If you are a sufferer and don't ever occasionally feel like this one then you probably won't ever feel like any of the others. It is the one which probably best fits the general description of how a depressed person might feel on any given day. They are in the "water" and sub-consciously "bobbing up and down" with the "waves" in their brain over which they have no control. Their brain is subconsciously trying to deal with it.

For many depressed people, on most days the "waves" might be the equivalent of only inches (centimetres) high. That would fine and no problem at all. A "depressed person" would be having a great day! On other days when the "waves" might be a bit higher it can begin to affect their ability to think about the normal day to day issues.

For the sufferer it's just enough to make them and their brain aware that the "sea" in their brain isn't calm any more and that it has to give some of their subconscious attention to dealing with it. As the "waves" grow in height it seems to me that your brain starts to progressively close down its' ability to deal **consciously** with anything other than how you are feeling and how your **subconscious** brain is dealing with it.

I know that there are various degrees of depression and I also know there are millions of people who are much more seriously affected than I am. However, I'd be surprised if other sufferers couldn't relate to how I feel in relation to the "sea analogy".

Certainly all of the sufferers I have spoken with do understand and some of them have said that is **"exactly how I feel"**.

For those with serious depression the "waves" in the "sea" inside their brain can be so high they reach the point where they become tired of trying to "mentally survive" and waiting to "mentally drown" and that they want to physically "end it all" instead.

I know that most non-sufferers can't understand a sufferers "need to end it all". More than one person has told me that it is both selfish and unthinkable for a sufferer to "end it all" when they are surrounded by people who love them and want to help them. But I **can** and really **DO** understand why people do end it all.

Even though I don't regard my self as a seriously depressed person I have been at that "end point" many times during my life even from as early as 13 years old when I can first remember wanting to die because of the way I felt. I've never actually done anything but I can remember thinking about it, being only a few seconds away from doing something about it and pulling back. Not just once but more times than I care to admit. In recent years it is only the thoughts of my family and friends which has stopped me. Ironically, at other times, they have been the cause of my depression.

The important thing I need you to remember here about the "Sea Wave" analogy is that it is almost entirely independent of everything else. When you wake up the "Sea Waves" in your brain are either small or large. There is nothing a sufferer can do to guarantee to improve it. Not then or at any time later during the day. The "Sea Waves" are a product of whatever is going on in your brain.

However, what happens in the other Dimensions can certainly make the "Sea Waves" **worse.** Nothing that happens in the other Dimensions can necessarily make it better. But, quite often, the "Sea Waves" and the other Dimensions do get better as the day progresses.

What typically happens when things get worse is that something causes a problem in one of the other Dimensions and this causes the "height" of the "Sea Waves" to increase. More than any other Dimension, the "Sea Wave" is a consequence of all of the others and the overall measure of how ill you feel. And it is the one over which you have least control.

This is perhaps the shortest explanation for any of the Dimensions because it is, arguably, the easiest to explain. Short though it may be, it describes the main feeling you get when you are depressed and it can easily be the worst. And, far more than the others, it is the one you almost always have a sense of feeling at any time of the day or night. So, coping with it is not something you can switch on and off as the need arises. You actually have to "cope" with it **ALL** of the time.

It's as if you have another job or another life in addition to the one you already have. And coping with it is not a part time job even though at times you don't feel too bad and you might say "I can cope with it easily". Coping with it is still a full time "job".

Let's now look at the next important Dimension. It is the one which **MOST** affects the "Sea Wave" (Dimension 1) and how you feel at any given point in time. It is called the "River Current". But before we move on I will summarise here in a few words the most important things I would like you to remember about this Dimension. I will add a Summary to the end of the other Dimensions too.

Summary.

- **Dimension 1** is the "Sea Wave" and is the main Dimension. It is the first and most important of the Red feelings. This relates to the overall feeling of Depression and is perhaps both the cause and the consequence of all of the others. It is the one over which a sufferer has no control. It's the way their brain is working when they wake up and nothing they can do during the day will necessarily make it better. **It may get better on its' own but, typically, the other Dimensions can only make it worse.**

4 - Dimension 2 – River Current
Red

- *This refers mostly to the feelings of Duty and Responsibility.*

This is the one feeling which is mostly a reflection of what happens to a sufferer during their day or what may have happened to them in the preceding days. It also best describes how people with depression are affected by **Duty and Responsibility** and how the turbulence of daily life and responsibilities can make them feel worse. It is the second of the Red feelings.

Knowing that a sufferer **HAS** to do things when they may not feel well enough to do them can sometimes make life seem unbearable for them. When you talk to someone who is medically qualified they often talk about levels of Anxiety. I believe it is the "River Current" which relates to the feelings of Anxiety. And it is the feeling which many people associate with Panic Attacks.

Using a new "water based analogy" now of a River and not the Sea, on a good day for the sufferer the "River" will be gently rippling over the rocks. It hardly moves and their subconscious brain is happily coping with the fact that as far as "mentally drowning" is concerned they are "on the surface and hardly moving" so things are under control. Their subconscious brain is dealing with it quietly and they are not consciously aware of it.

Now, imagine that instead of a slow moving river the sufferer is now in a kayak and "shooting the rapids" on a white water river in a canyon. The kayak they are in is being buffeted from side to side and the water is moving at about 40 miles per hour (65 kilometres per hour). Suddenly they fall out and are starting to drown. It isn't just the up and down motion of the waves that is affecting them most now, it is the speed at which they are being spun around and lashed against the rocks and then washed away.

The "River Currents" of daily life can affect a sufferers' ability to deal with even the simplest of tasks. Their brain during a depression can be seriously affected by the demands of daily life and they may be unable to cope with it. It often coincides with other demands made on them by family, friends and their job. Their **subconscious** brain tries to deal with it but the more it has to deal with then the less the sufferer feels able to deal with their **conscious** everyday issues.

The demands placed on them can escalate. The seriousness of the demands can increase too. As the deadlines loom ever closer and their ability to meet the challenges decreases this causes the "speed" of the "River Current" to increase too. And, as their conscious brain tries to deal with the day to day problems, their subconscious brain seems like it is using up far more of their brains apparent "total capacity". They have to work harder consciously to overcome the apparent reduced level of brain power to deal with things.

As this becomes an ever increasing problem for the sufferer it begins to affect the size of the "Sea Waves". So, not only is their brain trying not to let them "mentally drown" by being swept away at great speed by the "River Current" (Dimension 2), it is also trying not to let them "mentally drown" by the ever increasing size of the "Sea Waves" (Dimension 1).

Now imagine if something suddenly happens, typically when it seems to you as if things couldn't get worse, where a member of the family reminds you of something really critically important which you promised to do today. Or your Manager at work says he needs you to finish something extremely important which you should have done days ago but you haven't even had time to start it yet.

Suddenly, because the speed of the "River Current" (Dimension 2) is so great and the sufferer is hardly able to cope with what they are already trying to do, the size of the "Sea Waves" (Dimension 1) becomes huge. The sufferer suddenly can't cope any more as their brain struggles to keep them "mentally alive". It's then that they really know the feeling of depression. It's then that they reach their limit. I think people say it's when they have a Panic Attack and "hit the wall".

What makes things worse is that in their day to day life they will always be torn at the very same time in several different directions by family, friends and their work. It's like the river is always moving them in different directions and at widely differing speeds. The "River Current" (Dimension 2) may be taking them at great speed in one direction and their brain is already struggling to cope with that when this new priority might demand that they move immediately in a new and different direction but **at the same time** as they are still going in the old direction. They have to try and do both.

This new direction is almost certainly against the flow so if they are already "drowning" because they are being sucked in one direction, imagine how hard it is to desperately try to swim against the flow while also trying not to "drown". The "River Current" (Dimension 2) is the one which is most usually the cause of a bad day. If the sufferer already starts the day with a high "Sea Wave" (Dimension 1) then a rapidly increasing "River Current" as in Dimension 2 will come close to "finishing them off".

What their family and friends or manager at work do not know is how they feel at the point in time when they throw in that new challenge. How could they? And even if the sufferer told them, how could they explain it? Even if they did, most family and friends or colleagues have absolutely no concept of what it is like to be in the process of "mentally drowning". Why should they?

When family and friends throw in this new challenge or change of course they have every expectation that the sufferer will deal with it just as if they were completely well. And if the sufferer doesn't deal with it they are either offended or shocked. You can "imagine" people saying to the sufferer .....

..."What happened? Why didn't you do it? It was obvious what had to be done and when it had to be done by? All you needed to do was ...!"

I describe moments like this when family and friends or colleagues at work add sudden challenges to a sufferers' day as very much like them **"throwing bucket loads of water on an already drowning man"**. This is how I came up with the idea for the title of the book because most sufferers say they really indentify with this feeling and almost every day of their lives they have to cope with the "buckets of water".

Friends, family and colleagues at work have no idea how difficult it is for a sufferer to get their brain to quickly grasp and deal with this new challenge when their brain is already pre-occupied with varying levels of subconscious "mental survival". Failure to respond immediately in a positive way is often seen by the family and friends as being unhelpful or stupid. But they are the ones "throwing the bucket loads of water on the already drowning man".

It's not that they don't care but that they just **CAN'T** understand. And, most importantly, the sufferer often can't understand **either.** The sufferer just increasingly feels like a failure. The more like a failure they feel then the higher the "Sea Waves" (Dimension 1) become until they reach a point when the sufferer no longer wants to "mentally survive".

Quite often it is family or friends who unintentionally make the "River Current" (Dimension 2) worse as a result of which the "Sea Waves" (Dimension 1) increase to the point where the sufferer really doesn't want the "mental drowning" to go on for a second longer. Unintentionally, they tip the sufferer over the edge.

At work there is a difficult choice to make as to how honest a sufferer is about how they feel. Because there is so little understanding about depression it isn't something they can really "come clean" about. Consequently, time spent at work doing a job while also dealing with a rapid "River Current" (Dimension 2) and increasing "Sea Waves" (Dimension 1) can make a sufferer extremely tired in a way that sleep alone will never cure. (I will deal with sleep later in Chapter 13 – "Some other things to think about - especially family and friends").

There is nothing a sufferer can do to get out of the routine at work without it looking odd and someone coming up with the diagnosis that they aren't coping. Keeping it hidden when you are unwell is **FAR** more tiring than just doing the job. Doing both at the same time is often almost impossible and requires huge levels of effort.

So, the "River Current" (Dimension 2) is the one which is most easily affected by external situations and it is almost certainly the one which causes people with depression to avoid duty and responsibility and to lock themselves away and ignore what is going on around them. If you had been "mentally drowning" day after day and year after year wouldn't you want to find somewhere to hide where the day to day problems don't occur and you no longer felt that you were being washed away? If you could find a rock pool in a quiet bit of the "river" to hide in for a while you would seize it wouldn't you? When people are badly depressed, they look for that bit of calm water every minute of the day but they never seem to find it.

Once again let me summarise here the main points about this Dimension.

Summary.

- **Dimension 2** is the "River Current" and the next most serious feeling. It is the second Red feeling. I believe it is the "River Current" which most relates to the feelings of Anxiety. And it is the feeling which many people associate with Panic Attacks. It is the one which reflects a sufferers' daily life and, because it is the one which they can sometimes do something about, it can often be the reason why they hide away. **Adding to the sufferers' problems is like throwing bucket loads of water on an already drowning man.**

5 - Dimension 3 – Lake Shore

Red

- *This refers mostly to the feelings of Isolation and Vulnerability.*

When I first began developing this Model, I originally thought Dimension 3 – "Lake Shore" was the straight forward Dimension. That it would be the easiest Dimension to explain. But the more time I have had to think about it, the more I have realised that it really covers much more than I originally thought.

This is the one feeling where family and friends and the "Professionals" such as Doctors, Psychiatrists and Counsellors have most impact. Or perhaps as a result of their work in the other Dimensions, the sufferer feels the benefit most in this Dimension.

And using the "water based analogy" here, I want you to think about a lake. This lake I am asking you to imagine is a big lake where only on a clear day can you see the hills and shore on the other side. And although the waves on the surface of this lake may never be very big compared to the sea, if you are in the water in the middle of the Lake you can still be a long way from the shore where you might find help.

So, the "Lake Shore" (Dimension 3) is all about how close to safety you feel you are; as you try to overcome this feeling of "mentally drowning". It is a measure of the "distance the sufferer is from the Lake Shore or the safety of dry land". The distance from the Lake Shore refers to the feelings of **Isolation and Vulnerability.** It is the third and final Red feeling.

Now don't forget, in this "water based analogy" the depressed person **NEVER** gets out of the water but often they seek the comfort of knowing there is something or someone nearby which they can "mentally" hold onto or be supported by. You can imagine how important that can be, particularly to someone who is suffering and doesn't know what to do.

Because this Dimension is a bit more complex I am going to divide it into 3 parts which explain the different ways in which this feeling "works".

First – how close a sufferer feels to the "Lake Shore" and dry land is very much an indicator of how much support they are getting from the family and friends around them or from their Doctor, Psychiatrist or Counsellor. If it is good support then they know they don't have far to go to get help and that they will feel better once they get there. Let me be clear on this point too that it isn't the **amount** of support they are getting that makes them feel closer to the safety of land but the **quality.**

Let me explain what I mean by "quality".

You can have lots of people who claim to be supportive but if they don't understand what they are doing then they are almost certainly not helping at all. If the support the sufferer is getting isn't relevant or if their family and friends just don't understand then the sufferer might just as well be miles (kilometres) away from the "Lake Shore" and dry land. Getting the **right people** to give the sufferer the **right help** is critically important because it offers them that small bit of respite while they attempt to reduce the feeling of "mentally drowning".

Second – if the support the sufferer is getting isn't relevant or it is actually making things worse, then they are quite likely to "swim away from the Lake Shore" to stop people "throwing the buckets of water on them". If they are struggling to cope and the help isn't working then they will do whatever they can to avoid it because their brain is already fully occupied dealing with things in the best way it can. A sufferers' brain can't cope with help that is either irrelevant or actually damaging. It makes things **much** worse.

Third - this one is quite difficult to explain because it deals with contrary feelings at the same time. For example, sufferers often feel the need to be close to people (even if they are just in the next room) but they don't want to actually be in the **SAME** room

with them. Sufferers often say that they can get quite frightened when they feel they are getting a bit remote from people but, and this may sound odd, they also say they can get just as frightened when they are with them.

I suppose it is the security of knowing help might be there from people if they need it but it is tempered with the fear that these people might make things worse and "throw some buckets of water on them".

It is often best for a sufferer to get away and sit on their own in a public area such as a café knowing they are surrounded by people they don't know and have no need to meet. They know that these strangers are there to offer help if the sufferer needs or asks for it but that these other people are unlikely to make things worse because they are have no reason to ask the sufferer to do something that requires them to do it now and perform something they don't want to or feel able to do.

If it does turn out that these strangers can affect the sufferer then they can leave or "swim away from the Lake Shore" and maybe find another "rock pool" where they can rest.

The "Lake Shore" (Dimension 3) is all about the sufferers' need for or how close they feel to safety or support. Or a measure of the quality of the support they are getting. If they aren't getting any support or what they are getting isn't working it has the effect of pushing the sufferer away from the safety of the "Lake Shore" and land.

Sufferers often feel isolated and remote from the real world and the people whom they love and those who love them. Even though they may be surrounded by love, it may not be enough to bring them "closer to the Lake Shore and land".

Only when family and friends understand them and what affects them in their attempts to avoid this permanent and, at times, intolerable and exhausting "mental drowning" can they really feel that they are nearer to the "Lake Shore" and land.

So, the message for loved ones, family and friends is this; even though it can be one of the most difficult things for them to understand, there may be times for sufferers when **all the love in the world may not be enough to help them.** It may not be what the sufferer needs and, what is worse, the provider of that love and support may become disillusioned, hurt and distant because they think the sufferer doesn't want their love or support.

It is important that the family and friends understand that sufferers **DO** want their love and support even if they may not appear to realise or appreciate it.

Sometimes love and support doesn't necessarily make them feel better or "closer to the Lake Shore" which is what they really need. That may be because the sufferer may not understand what they need and so they can't communicate it effectively to those closest to them. And what the sufferer thinks they want isn't always what they **need. "Wants"** are very different to **"needs".**

Now, at the risk of being politically incorrect here, I do believe that having people around is more likely to be of help to women than to men. Apparently, women prefer to talk about their problems whereas it seems that men tend not to.

So, a man may disappear off to be alone in an effort to get "closer to the Lake Shore". But women are more likely to meet up with family and friends and talk in an effort for them to get "closer to the Lake Shore".

In this sense I believe there is a fundamental difference with depression between men and women. It's just my view and I claim no scientific reason for it. Interestingly, most of the sufferers I have spoken with agree with "my theory".

So, in the "Lake Shore" (Dimension 3), I believe women are more likely to swim **TO** the "Lake Shore" and men are more likely to swim **AWAY** from it.

Perhaps the excellent and very entertaining book called "Men are from Mars, Women are from Venus" by Dr. John Gray (ISBN 0-5833-4499-2) will explain it better than I can.

Now in much the same way that the three principle physical Dimensions in science are length, width and height, I believe that the first three Dimensions I have described are the three main ones to do with depression.

Some of the sufferers I have spoken with feel the "Lake Shore" (Dimension 3) might be compared to the stress levels they feel. I prefer to see it as a measure of Isolation and Vulnerability. It is Dimension 8 – Rain which I feel most closely fits the feeling of Stress.

Now, here is the Summary.

Summary.

- **Dimension 3** is the "Lake Shore" and is a measure of how good the support is or how sufferers benefit from the help their family and friends, and Professionals including Counsellors give them. The "Lake Shore" refers to the feelings of Isolation and Vulnerability. It is the third and final Red feeling. The distance from the "Lake Shore" is a measure of how isolated or vulnerable they feel and, subject to the quality of the support, they will either swim towards the shore or away from it. Family and friends need to understand how to get the sufferer to "swim towards them". They also need to understand that whatever they do and however hard they try to help, the sufferer just may not be able to swim any closer. **To the sufferer, all the love in the world may not be enough to help them at that time.**

6 - Dimension 4 – Time

Amber

- *This mostly refers to the feeling of Need for or the Benefit of Support.*

Just like in Dimension 3 - "Lake Shore", there are three ways of looking at Dimension 4. Firstly, Time can be a measure of the length of time overall that a sufferer has been suffering with depression or, secondly, it can be a measure of how long they have felt unwell or at a particular level. But there is a third way which can be even more important. "Time" relates to the feelings of **"Need for"** or the **"Benefit of Support"**. It is the first of the Amber (Yellow) feelings.

Because this Dimension is also a bit more complex, let's explore each one for a moment.

First – if, like me, the sufferer has been suffering from depression for many years, there is a feeling in some people, such as family and friends, that it can't possibly have been that bad for you because you have coped for all of this time. That is a difficult argument to defend. But the reality is you just carry on because you have to and don't know what else to do.

Sufferers learn to hide from others how they feel but the length of time they suffer with it definitely doesn't make it any easier. And, at times, the longer they have had it makes it all the harder to deal with. They just wish it would end and they could get on with things.

Let's not forget that, as I have coped for many years, one could argue that I have been relatively lucky. Some sufferers don't cope and it incapacitates them to such an extent and for such a length of time that they have no choice but to submit themselves to a much higher level of intervention. I don't think I or they would describe the symptoms or the feelings differently but the intensity of the feelings which other sufferers experience is clearly much greater than mine.

Second – the length of time that a particular episode of depression can last may vary from just a few hours to several months and even years. When my longest episode of several weeks ended then suddenly, within minutes and without any warning or obvious reason, I felt much better.

Not fully recovered but sufficiently improved to know that I felt better and to truly appreciate just how ill I had been before. There was a definite sense of relief because I suddenly felt I could relax, if only for a moment. It felt as though I had reached a shallow pool where I could rest for a while.

For most of the time while I was really ill I had been in a serious "Sea Wave" (Dimension 1) and "River Current" (Dimension 2) environment where the levels of intensity had hardly ever changed. As a result I really felt the distance from the "Lake Shore" (Dimension 3) was huge and I was miles (kilometres) from safety and support even though it was never far away.

Now, on some occasions the length of time a sufferer feels depressed can have a big impact on how long it takes to improve. And yet on other occasions, such as the one I've just mentioned, the change can be dramatic and quick. I can find no logic to the way it works but, the length of time the sufferer is unwell is quite likely to have a direct effect on how long it takes to recover. Many sufferers I have spoken with have experienced the same thing.

During any given day, how a sufferer feels can change several times. It may be in response to external things (which primarily affect the "River Current" - Dimension 2) or the way they feel as a vulnerable person (the "Lake Shore" - Dimension 3). It can be helpful for a sufferer to track their mood changes to see how they are doing.

I believe it is now possible for me at any time of the day or night to assess how I feel "numerically" and, if you are a sufferer, you will begin to understand this when you complete the Self Assessment Chart in Appendix 1 at the end of the book.

Third – and perhaps **MOST** importantly, it can be the time a sufferer spends with other people in their company and the effect they have on them. And here I need to make a distinction because people fall broadly into 2 categories:-

- People whose company a sufferer **HAS** to be in at any given time and for any prescribed length of time. Typically these are work colleagues and family with whom they live.

- People whose company a sufferer **CHOOSES** to be in at a time that suits them and meets their needs. These are typically friends but can also mean family when they deliberately set out to spend time with them for the purpose of enjoying their company. It obviously includes Professionals such as Doctors, Psychiatrists and Counsellors too.

Let's have a closer look at each of these groups.

Colleagues - let's begin by considering the role of work colleagues.

Clearly, a sufferer spends a lot of time with their work colleagues but they are the least likely to have a **positive** impact on a sufferers feelings. Sufferers may not have a choice in their job as to how much of their working day they spend in the company of colleagues and so they may have to act out their part as best they can while trying to overcome some very intense feelings as they do.

It is important for a sufferer to understand that their colleagues have their own jobs and issues to deal with and, while they may like them and want to help if they can, the motivation for them to do anything significant to help a sufferer is low. Experience will tell you that to rely on them is not sensible for the sufferer and could equally be "very unfair" on their colleagues.

Family – now family are different. Let's now consider their role.

Sufferers often live with family and, to a greater or lesser extent, depending how much they understand about how the sufferer feels or the degree to which family are supportive, sufferers will enjoy that time or it will add to their feeling of depression.

I don't believe that any family member would consciously set out deliberately to make a sufferer feel worse (other than in exceptional circumstances) but because they are busy and have their own lives to lead, of which the sufferer is only a part, sometimes family can't be of much help and that can have a big impact on how a sufferer feels.

Families have the greatest potential to try and make things better or actually make things worse. And whichever it is will affect the amount of time the depressed person feels able to spend in the company of family.

If the sufferer **doesn't** enjoy spending a long time in their company but the family is positively motivated to help, then together they need to find out why and how to improve things.

If the family is being helpful and the depressed person **does** enjoy the help they give then it is perhaps **even more important** to find out **why** so that they don't lose whatever it is that makes the difference.

Friends - now let's consider the role of Friends

Friends can sometimes be of far more help than family and if not handled correctly it can cause the family to feel offended. And the reason for the difference has to do with duty and responsibility (Dimension 2).

Do you remember the analogy in the Chapters that dealt with "River Current" (Dimension 2) and the "Lake Shore" (Dimension 3) and how they impacted on a sufferers' daily life. They were often some of the main reasons for swimming away from the "Lake Shore" to avoid the feeling of duty and responsibility because that adds to the pressure sufferers feel. And that makes them feel worse.

One of the main reasons why friends, and in this case I also include Doctors, Psychiatrists and Professional Counsellors, can be of most help is because the time sufferers spend with them is relatively short and is usually arranged at a time that meets their needs. They help by spending time with the sufferer with the specific objective, expressed or otherwise, of taking their mind off how they feel or exploring ways to improve things. There is typically less pressure, responsibility and duty to do anything.

However, where family is concerned, there is a permanent and often deeply felt sense of duty and responsibility in the sufferer towards the family which can cast a shadow over everything else. It quietly adds to the height of the "Sea Wave" (Dimension 1) and can easily lead to the "River Current" (Dimension 2) increasing rapidly with no warning.

So, there is always a "tension" with family, however small that might be, which is far less likely to occur when you are in the company of friends or Doctors, Psychiatrists and Professional Counsellors.

I don't mean to imply here that sufferers do not respect the time they spend with friends or Doctors, Psychiatrists and Professional Counsellors, or that they lack any feeling of duty or responsibility to them but that the relationship is different. Good friends will understand that. Doctors, Psychiatrists and Counsellors know it.

So for the benefit of family in particular I need to explain that the reason a sufferer may choose friends over family at any given time is not because they don't love you or appreciate the help you give them on a daily basis but because they sometimes gain more by spending some time with friends where their deep sense of duty and responsibility is not involved in or affects the "temporary healing process".

Summary.

- **Dimension 4** is "Time". "Time" relates to the feelings of "Need for" or the "Benefit of Support". It is the first of the Amber (Yellow) feelings. It can refer to the time they have suffered with depression or even how long a depressive episode can last. But mostly it refers to the time sufferers spend with people and how family, friends and work colleagues can have a widely differing effect on helping them feel better. Even the closest family member may not be the best person to help. Sometimes, duty and responsibility towards family makes it more difficult. **The best help comes from people a sufferer chooses to be with.**

7 - Dimension 5 – Temperature

Amber

- *This refers mostly to the feeling of Despair.*

In this metaphorical "water based analogy" I am using, where I compare how someone might feel as if they were "drowning", then the way in which I feel the temperature might be used is as a measure of the depth of despair that all sufferers feel when they are unwell.

In every day temperatures go up and down and so does a sufferers' feeling of despair. And despair is caused by the feeling of being unable to resolve how you feel or get out of the situation in which you find yourself. So "Temperature" relates to the level of your feelings of **Despair.** It is the second of the Amber (Yellow) feelings.

If you have always lived in a hot climate then it might be difficult to imagine what it is like to feel cold. To feel so cold that you can't stop shivering. To be in the cold sea knowing there is nothing to protect you from the cold water. To feel so cold that you feel the cold has "penetrated" your bones. But for most people they can imagine how that feels. If not, place your hand in some ice/iced water for a short while but not for too long as it could harm your hand

Well, on a bad day, in addition to all of the other things that are happening to a sufferer, it can feel as if the despair is so great it has penetrated to the very core of your being. Nothing can improve it quickly. And, as a sufferer, **YOU** don't seem to be able to change it at all. You just know you are "in the cold water" and you can't get out.

So, in addition to the "Sea Waves" (Dimension 1) and the "River Current" (Dimension 2) and the "Lake Shore" (Dimension 3) and the "Time" (Dimension 4) you always have to somehow cope with the "Temperature" (Dimension 5) too.

Now on some days the temperature of the "water" does not have a negative effect on a sufferer. It can be likened to "luke warm" and quite pleasant. On a few days it can even be "very warm" like bath water and almost exhilarating. But the temperature is **never** something that makes the sufferer, metaphorically, want to stay in the water.

In the same way, on some days the despair can be huge (as if the water was very cold) and they struggle to survive it. On other days they may not feel particularly despondent but a sufferer will know that they aren't happy (as if the water was luke warm). On some days a sufferer may feel happy (as if the water was comfortably hot) even though they know it is a temporary respite from how they might feel soon.

Part of the act which most sufferers have to occasionally "put on" is to appear happy for the benefit of family, friends or those they work with. On a typical day that is a bit like saying to their family, friends and colleagues that "the water is hot and lovely" even though they feel it is only luke warm. Imagine them trying to tell family and friends that the water is "hot and lovely" when they actually feel it is "freezing cold" and the cold has "penetrated" their bones.

If you were in the water and freezing cold then everyone would be able to see you shivering and that you looked cold. In much the same way, no matter how hard they might try, there is no way when a sufferer has a deep feeling of despair during a depressive episode that they can successfully persuade others they are OK.

And most important of all, Dimension 5 has the greatest effect on the three main Dimensions. It is most unlikely that a sufferer will feel alright in Dimension 1 (the "Sea Wave"), Dimension 2 (the "River Current") or Dimension 3 (the "Lake Shore") if they don't feel well in Dimension 5 (the "Temperature").

At times like this the family, friends and colleagues around you want you to be happy and will often do whatever they can to lift your spirits. But if the cold of the despair has penetrated to the very core of your being, then it may take a sufferer a long time to recover.

And what is difficult for a sufferer to explain to others is that their ability to lift themselves out of despair may not even be within their control. Sometimes, it doesn't matter how hard they try, they can't change how they feel. Worse still there are some days when a sufferer doesn't even have the energy or the motivation to even try.

The problem with those days is that it is very hard for the family, friends, work colleagues and those others around the sufferer to know how to deal with them. On the one hand they don't like seeing them like this and want to help and, on the other, it annoys them that the sufferer is casting a dark shadow over "their" day particularly if, in spite of all of their well meaning efforts, nothing seems to work.

Depending at that time on the temperament of the people around a sufferer, they can be supportive in a way that is helpful or they can be impatient and obstructive to anything the sufferer is trying to do for themselves. Then, to you the sufferer, Dimension 3 – "Lake Shore" comes to your rescue and you metaphorically drift or "swim away from the Lake Shore" to find some warmer water and some inner peace.

Ironically, during periods of despair, having people around you can be helpful but that may well depend on the people and the environment you are all in. If it is primarily social then a sufferer has the best possible situation to help improve their mood. But if it is work or there are things to be done and the people around them are expecting the sufferer to join in, regardless of how they feel, it can be very difficult.

Typically, if you are depressed, then people make your despair worse not better.

For the most part, because a feeling of despair can last all day, or even several days, getting away from people is often the best plan for a sufferer. However, because the "Lake Shore" (Dimension 3) makes you feel more vulnerable the further you are away from the "Lake Shore", it isn't a good idea for a sufferer to create **TOO** big a distance between themselves and other people. Often the best plan is for them to go back to bed and just sleep through it. To non-sufferers that may seem very odd!

I find that I need to do the same thing. I don't find sitting quietly in a chair in a room on my own or even lying down is enough. I have to go to sleep even if it is only for a few minutes.

Now this can't really happen in a "work environment" because few workplaces provide beds. But even with family and friends, they often find it very difficult to understand why the sufferer feels the need to go back to bed. As far as they are concerned they are being lazy or anti-social. Family and friends don't realise that it may be the best option to get a sufferer through what may be a very difficult period of time for them.

It has often been said to me, "Why don't you go for a walk?" On some days when you are depressed it can be very helpful but if it is also mixed with despair it can be "dangerous". For sufferers who are "on the edge of their tolerance" for what they are experiencing, adding distance from the "Lake Shore" and increasing their vulnerability could add to their problems.

As an example of this (and until I had analysed this feeling), I could never understand why on two consecutive days in similar weather a few years ago I went on exactly the same walk and on the first day came back feeling much better yet on the second day I had to abandon the walk and come home. Only now do I realise that on the first day I didn't have a deep feeling of despair whereas on the second day I remember that I did.

So despair can be a very big factor in a sufferer's ability to cope with everything else that is going on. It has the biggest impact on the other Dimensions. Helping someone out of a feeling of despair can be difficult and sometimes it isn't possible.

At times like that, all you can do is make sure they are safe and let them come through it themselves.

Summary.

- **Dimension 5** is "Temperature". So "Temperature" relates to the level of a sufferers' feeling of Despair. It is the second but perhaps most important of the Amber (Yellow) feelings. It is a broad measure of despair and the lower the temperature then the deeper is the despair. While a sufferer can try and lift themselves out of this feeling sometimes it just isn't possible. And while family, friends and colleagues at work may try to help, at the end of the day, only they can achieve it. **And much to the annoyance of those around the sufferer, on some days they neither can nor want to.**

8 - Dimension 6 – Pressure

Amber

- *This refers mostly to the feeling of Motivation.*

Continuing with our "water based analogy" of the sufferer "mentally drowning", you may wonder where pressure fits in?

Let me ask you to think about a "barometer" for a moment. A barometer measures the atmospheric pressure. You can often find a barometer hanging on someones' living room wall or in the hallway just inside the front door. It is used to give an indication when the weather is changing.

We are most used to seeing references to changing atmospheric pressure during Television weather forecasts that we see, either before or after the news. The presenters often talk about "low pressure fronts" and what happens when the "atmospheric pressure is high".

Put simply:-

- Low pressure means

  storms and low clouds, heavy rain and high winds.

- High pressure means

  cloudless skies, higher than average temperatures, no wind.

Or to put this even more simply:-

- Low pressure means

  Bad weather

- High pressure means

  Good weather

In my multi-Dimensional analysis of the feelings associated with depression I compare "Pressure" (Dimension 6) to the feeling of **Motivation** within the sufferer. Motivation might be described as an inner feeling of "pressure to do something". It is the third of the Amber (Yellow) feelings.

Some people regard this Dimension or feeling in people who suffer with depression as a form of apathy. But, before we go any further, I need to express my own personal distinction here.

Apathy is where people **aren't inclined to do anything.**

I don't believe that is true about sufferers with depression. They are typically not apathetic people by nature so I prefer to think of it as low Motivation. People who are depressed are typically people who, were it not for the depression or even in spite of it, are highly motivated. Remember, depressed people are often high achievers and successful people. Apathetic people rarely achieve anything.

Low Motivation can occur because of the way a sufferer feels. And because of the way they feel there are times when they can't do anything about it. Typically, when they are "mentally drowning" with high and fast moving waves all around them their motivation to do anything else is low. During times when they don't feel so bad their motivation does come back to them.

However, and **this is important,** I don't think that sufferers with depression usually have consistently high motivation for any length of time. But their normal level of motivation may still be higher than average.

But when they do, it can be extremely high and much higher than for non-sufferers simply because "it has to be". Motivation requires a kind of effort and energy that sufferers don't always have ready to be used. When they do have to do something that, for them, requires "super human effort" then they behave a bit like a weight lifter.

If you can imagine any of the impressive weight lifters in the Olympics, they walk onto a mat carrying absolutely nothing then **suddenly** walk up to a metal bar on the floor in front of them with very large and heavy round weights attached to each end and lift the bar high above their head. They hold it there for only as long as necessary to qualify as "a lift".

As soon as they don't need to hold the bar high above their heads any longer they drop it and walk away. And unless they absolutely have to, they don't want to come back and try it again. They have done their "bit", achieved "the lift" and that is it. More importantly, most other people may not have been able to lift that heavy weight and achieve it at all.

A sufferer with depression acts in much the same way.

They often do things in shorter periods of "higher energy". Even if they are feeling really ill with high "Sea Waves" (Dimension 1), strong "River Current" (Dimension 2) and a significant distance from the "Lake Shore" (Dimension 3) they may often achieve something incredible for themselves which non-sufferers may just see as "normal" but which for the sufferer is nothing short of a miracle.

Or they might suddenly achieve something so great no-one understands how they did it because it exceeded every-ones' expectations and no-one else they know could have done it.

Some of the worlds' cleverest and most successful people suffer(ed) with depression. People like Sir Winston Churchill during World War 2 who is widely regarded as one the Worlds' greatest ever leaders.

And I feel sure that "high achieving sufferers" like him would understand exactly what I am about to tell you.

I remember an occasion vividly which for me at the time was a great "weight-lifting experience". What is it that I did for myself which at the time required such "super human" effort from me?

I made myself a cup of coffee. That's all I did.

And it took me 30 minutes because I had to keep stopping and restarting. But it was the first one I felt well enough to make myself for over 2 weeks. And I did feel better once I had done it. But to be honest, I felt like I had run up a steep and dangerous hill in the dark for over an hour. I was mentally and physically exhausted.

Prior to that, no matter how hard I tried, and even though I knew at times I wanted it, I couldn't motivate myself to go and make it. Succeeding was a huge achievement for me.

Now, when you hear someone describe their inability to do something as simple as making a cup of coffee, when previously they have been used to managing people and large Multi-million dollar budgets sometimes for major Banks and working Internationally across the world, where failure to make things work to cost and on time is absolutely unthinkable, you have to ask yourself why didn't they just get up and do it?

Well I can't answer that. I just know that if I could have done it I would.

But at the time I did know that I felt too unwell (my sub-conscious was dealing with all of the "waves" and "currents" in my brain and my subconscious efforts to avoid "mentally drowning") that I did not believe that I had any spare capacity of brain power left to achieve it. The effort required was just too much. I wasn't even sure at the time if I could remember how to make a cup of coffee anyway.

So Motivation is very definitely affected by depression but, at times and with "super human effort", sufferers can motivate themselves to do things that they might not think possible to achieve at the time but which to the non-sufferer may seem hardly worth even thinking about because it only takes two minutes.

Some people think sufferers are lazy but it isn't laziness that stops them from doing everything they are asked. They often lack the confidence but also feel an almost constant and overwhelming need to save their effort by not doing anything when they are unwell so that they **CAN** do something later. Experience tells the sufferer that doing something now could make them too mentally exhausted to achieve or understand how to do something later which might be quite simple.

Depression can cause the sufferer to be associated with low output. That is clearly not very good at work or at home. So, to avoid that, the sufferer often has to work exceptionally hard at work and at home by motivating themselves to do things which their colleagues, family and friends may find no trouble at all.

And that "something" they have to do may actually be something very small and which is very simple.

So, after work and either before or when they get home, the sufferer is often exhausted and needs time to recover. Typically, women may seek the company of family and friends to unwind and men may lock themselves away. But both men and women are just trying to do the same thing; to get away from the duties and responsibilities they associate with work and home or the possibility that someone might "throw some buckets of water on them" so they can rebuild their motivation.

There is also another side to Motivation and that has to do with a feeling of purpose.

If one of the main reasons for someone getting up in the morning is taken away as in the case of the loss of a loved one or job, then it is very difficult for a sufferer to motivate themselves to do anything else. I think that is true for anyone but it is **particularly true** for someone with depression because the lack of purpose just adds to their depression and, as a result, it further lowers their Motivation.

Sometimes people with depression have to find a purpose, however small, in order to find some motivation for doing anything. But you can't replace "true purpose" with "artificial objectives".

It isn't that simple.

You can't give a sufferer things to do to "make them feel better" because it has the opposite effect to Motivation. It feels like "buckets of water are being thrown at them" and can make things worse.

To a sufferer it can even feel a bit like someone is fixing heavy lead weights to their legs as they try to stay afloat in the water.

Summary.

- **Dimension 6** is "Pressure" and is all about the feeling of Motivation (the inner pressure to do something). It is the third of the Amber (Yellow) feelings. Depression affects a sufferers' motivation. And if a sufferer has to motivate themselves to do even the simplest of tasks it can be absolutely exhausting. Expecting someone with depression to do things may not be realistic. It isn't that they are lazy but at times they lack the Motivation to do things that anyone else might do easily and without effort. Lack of purpose will make things worse. **Forcing sufferers to do things that they see no point in or don't feel able to do because of low Motivation can make their depression worse to the extent that they then increase the distance from the "Lake Shore" (Dimension 3) by swimming away from safety and support.**

9 - Dimension 7 – Wind

Amber

- *This refers mostly to the feeling of Confidence.*

In the analogy for this Dimension I would like you to think about the wind.

A wind can be anything from a light breeze that cools your face on a hot day to a violent storm with speeds up to 200 miles per hour (320 kilometres per hour) which demolishes buildings and whole communities. A light breeze may affect nothing more than a few butterflies but a violent storm can kill and destroy lives.

But whatever the strength of the wind, it represents movement and change. And people who suffer with depression do not like change. It's mostly because they create their own comfort or even "survival zones" around themselves and anything that changes that environment in which they manage to live represents a demand on them to do something which will accommodate that change.

And that requires effort and thinking, both precious resources that they may not have enough of when they are needed. So, "Wind" relates to the feelings associated with dealing with change such as

Confidence. It is the fourth and last of the Amber (Yellow) feelings.

So, how do we use a measure like the wind to explain how change affects a sufferer?

The way I describe it is that everyone, whether they suffer with depression or not, has an ability to be able to cope with or initiate change. Some days the ability may be very low, like the effect of a light breeze, yet on other days you can suggest huge change, like the effect of a very strong wind, and the person asked will even lead from the front.

In the past I have managed some major Multi-million dollar Change Programmes (these were the equivalent to violent storms for many people) and overcome significant internal and external opposition to ensure that the Project is successful.

So on some days, I might score 10 out of 10 for my confidence and ability to cope with, lead others and deal with change. But mostly, when I feel unwell, it will be closer to 3 or 4. It has occasionally been as low as 1 which on my scale is as low as it can get.

Let's not confuse Change with "Motivation" (Dimension 6).

You can be quite highly motivated but not feel comfortable with, or even want, the change. Or you can accept the change and yet not feel Motivated to do anything about it. So, while they are similar, they are definitely **different.**

And it is important to understand what happens when you force change on someone who suffers with depression. That could be as simple as asking them to do something quite simple when their confidence is low. This is very much the situation where the sufferer feels those "buckets of water crashing down on their heads". Change can force them to move from a situation where they have managed to find some inner peace and respite from the "mental drowning".

Typically, sufferers work at the same place with the same colleagues and go home just the same as they always do. They live with the same family and have the same friends. Everything stays the same.

But if the sufferer finds out that there is to be some major change in their lives such as their job is going to change and they have to take on much more responsibility or it even requires them to move to a new city and their family don't want to move, this would take the sufferer away from their existing and well established support structures.

You can see how a major change in circumstances would seriously affect their ability to cope. This would affect all of the main Dimensions with a big rise in the "Sea Wave" (Dimension 1) and a feeling they were being swept away by the "River Current" (Dimension 2). Having to move away from the support of their family and friends would severely increase their vulnerability hence the distance from the "Lake Shore" (Dimension 3) would increase whether they wanted it to or not.

If a sufferer is asked to do something relatively **SIMPLE** it can often feel to them just as bad as the major change I just described. I know that to non sufferers that can seem totally disproportionate. But it has to do with their confidence and sensitivity of their feelings at the time and especially the levels of intensity of feelings in the other Dimensions.

For example, asking a sufferer to do something as simple as making a cup of coffee could make them suddenly feel really ill with depression. How can you easily explain that to family, friends or colleagues at work?

Although I don't think I have ever felt this way, I do know that some sufferers are prone to respond aggressively to being asked to do the simplest of things. How do you explain a sufferers' violent reaction to a simple request by a relative or friend?

One of the other aspects of confidence to deal with Change is the element of risk associated with it.

If you are depressed then the very last thing you want to do is start anything that is likely to go wrong. You often lack the confidence to ensure that everything will go right. Mentally, you may have too many other issues to deal with and sorting out a mess which you might have inadvertently caused or just been part of is just too great a risk.

So, depression has the effect of reducing or even eliminating any sense of risk or adventure. This means that a sufferer can end up being stuck in a "rut". If they still had any confidence or sense of adventure in them, then doing something different might help to alleviate some of their feelings.

The apparent inability of a sufferer to do things could even explain why, when an opportunity presents itself to do something as simple and as pleasant as to go for a walk there is tendency just to stay at home. Not only is the Motivation not there but the sense of adventure, the confidence and willingness to experience change, no matter how small, is gone too.

It also has an impact on enjoyment and fun. Even sufferers who are passionate about hobbies and interests will stop doing them because they lack the enthusiasm. When I feel unwell, I stop reading books and listening to music, both of which I normally enjoy.

To use the wind analogy in a different way, it's as if you have been blown off course by the "wind". Things you would normally have the confidence to do but require that you go somewhere or do something just may not happen because it represents a change from your current comfort or survival zone, whatever that is and wherever that is.

Summary.

- **Dimension 7** is "Wind" and is all about Change. "Wind" relates to the feelings associated with change and a sufferers' ability to deal with it because of their level of confidence. It is the fourth and last of the Amber (Yellow) feelings. People who are depressed do not like change and have perhaps a higher than normal resistance to it. It is important to get some idea of a sufferers ability to cope with change as that can have a big affect on how they deal with it, and how that affects the other Dimensions, when change comes their way. Equally, sufferers avoid risk, even though they might not seem to care anymore. **Although sufferers might desperately want change for the better they fear change because for them it always seems to get worse or can make them feel ill.**

10 - Dimension 8 – Rain

Green

- *This refers mostly to the feeling of Stress.*

It may seem like I am repeating an analogy here because using my "water based analogy" I do keep referring to people throwing "buckets of water on an already drowning man" which might seem to have a similarity with "rainfall".

Clearly, if you are drowning, you have enough worries dealing with the water you are in. And my earlier remarks about how others may set you challenges that deeply affect you when they metaphorically "throw buckets of water over you" is aimed at immediate family and friends and what they may throw at you. Or even the challenges that your colleagues at work may throw at you.

Those are specific challenges given to you by **people you KNOW.**

But in this particular "water based analogy", I use Rain to describe challenges that may be given to you by **people you DON'T know.**

It's a "different kind of water" that represents the other things that are going on in your life over which you have little or **NO CONTROL.** It is the general feeling you get when things are not going well for you. "The Rain" relates to the feeling of **Stress**. It is the first of the Green feelings.

In much the same way that rain can be a fine drizzle that feels refreshing on your skin or it can be a downpour where several inches (centimetres) of water falls in a few minutes as a result of a storm, the wider effects of what is going wrong in your life can have a big impact.

Imagine coping with thunder and lightning, and the torrential rain in a storm while you are trying to avoid "drowning". To a sufferer it just makes what is already difficult seem impossible and even more unpleasant.

Some people seem to have all of the luck don't they? And then there are others who hardly seem to get any.

Have you ever heard the song "Don't let it Rain on my Parade" which was originally sung by Barbra Streisand in the 1964 film "Funny Girl"? Well some people go through a period in their life where it does rain a lot on "their Parade" and if they suffer with depression they find it more difficult to cope with than perhaps other people might.

I use this Dimension to get a feel of just how much is going wrong in a sufferer's life which is contributing negatively to how they feel. If it's raining on your Parade and you are a sufferer then the chances are you will struggle to cope with the effects they have on all of the other Dimensions.

Sometimes the cause of depression can be sat right in front of you. And having some form of measure of how good or bad your life seems to be to you at that time can be very helpful in working out what that is. And it can be caused by things over which you have no control.

So, you can begin to see how for some people who are struggling to survive the experience of "mentally drowning"; when they are already struggling to cope with Dimensions 1, 2, 3, 4, 5, 6 and 7, when they also have to cope with the external effects of "Rain" (Dimension 8), over which they have no control, as well it means there really is no-where to hide and get well.

In a strange way it has the effect of removing all of your choices.

It anchors you at a point far away from the "Lake Shore" (Dimension 3). You can't swim towards the "Lake Shore" or away from it. You can't swim in **any** direction. You can't respond to support because support won't change things. There are too many outside factors going wrong in your life and any time you spend trying to get help seems increasingly less likely to make any difference to you.

It is the equivalent of not being able to find any calm water on "your river" where you can find a few moments to rest. Or, even if you wanted to, you can't reach the "Lake Shore" because you are prevented from moving.

Often sufferers feel they are losing the battle with their depression when, in spite of their efforts and those of their family and friends, things happen to them which are outside of their control. This can seriously add to their levels of depression because nothing anyone can do will make a difference. "Rain" is often the cause where sufferers feel the need to "give up".

In addition to everything else, they **feel** powerless to make any changes even if they wanted to.

Summary.

Dimension 8 is "Rain" and is all about what is going on or wrong in a sufferers life. It may even be a measure of the subconscious issues that they have. "Rain" relates to the feeling of Stress. It is the first of the Green feelings. Is life difficult? If it is, then Dimension 8 is the place where a sufferer can take account of that feeling. And it is important to understand whether or not things are going well because it makes everything else so difficult if they are trying to cope and want to benefit from support. **When things around a sufferer are difficult it is a bit like being anchored miles (kilometres) from the "Lake Shore" and out of reach of the help they want and need.**

11 - Dimension 9 – Stars

Green

- *This refers mostly to the feelings of Memory Loss and Confusion.*

For the last 1,000 years, and probably for thousands of years before that, Sailors have used the Stars in the Night Sky to guide them to where they are going. Or just to help find out where they are.

If you are going to be permanently in the water, as you are in this "water based analogy", then part of the time in every 24 hours of your "day" will be night time. And, subject to how you are coping, you might get the chance to look up and look at the Stars.

When a sufferer is seriously depressed then they very rarely get the chance to think about anything else. Metaphorically "looking up at the sky" isn't an option. But the Stars in this analogy represent markers or memory points in their brain and the thousands of "mental routes" that they use to do things or get from A to B.

The difficulty with depression is that you forget very easily, both facts and the processes of how to do things. Your subconscious brain is fully occupied with avoiding the "mental drowning" and somehow it seems that your conscious brain, where you seem to remember these things, just wants to "power down". You can easily become very confused.

"Stars" relates to the feeling of **Memory Loss** and **Confusion**. It is the second of the Green feelings.

So when a sufferer is depressed and if they "metaphorically" look up at the "Stars" to remember how to do something or see the route from A to B, it seems to the sufferer that they can't see any Stars they recognise. Or they can't find the important Star that they urgently want now. All of the stars seem to be "clouded over". They have little or no power of recall.

For a sufferer this can be very embarrassing at home and potentially very difficult at work. At home it can also be very annoying for family and friends because sufferers no longer seem to have any grasp of what is going on around them and they have difficulty doing things they would normally do easily. Depending what kind of work they do, it can be dangerous for their own safety and the safety of others.

People may ask a sufferer to do things and even seconds later they will either completely forget or they can't remember how to do it. Or they will only partly remember and only partly do what they have agreed. What is worse is that they will probably forget how do something that is either very easy (like making a cup of coffee) that they have successfully done a thousand times before for most of their life.

Lists become essential and then the worst part for a sufferer is when they follow the list but forget to do something they should obviously have done at the same time but which was not on the list. Like going to the store for bread because the list says so but forgetting the milk because they forgot to put it on the list.

To a sufferer it seems like their subconscious brain slows the speed of the whole brain down until it can reach a point where things still work. But that speed is usually far too slow to enable them to function in the way that their job or their family and friends need them to. And that doesn't help their family, friends and work colleagues who may become very frustrated at how forgetful the sufferer has become. They can't rely on the sufferer any more.

And that is one of the most awful feelings to a sufferer when they know family and friends no longer trust them to be reliable. It really destroys their confidence and self esteem and seriously affects their willingness to even try to do things.

Now sometimes a sufferer won't have a problem and will be able to remember most things. But, their ability to use logic and process information does become less sound and, depending how ill they feel, increasingly it will let them down. What used to be easy for them suddenly becomes very difficult. And it causes them to become even more depressed about how forgetful they are becoming. It makes them very frustrated too.

But it isn't **JUST** their memory that is affected. It is the way they collect and process information too. As a result, they become reluctant to do anything because they become concerned that they may fail or look stupid. Or much worse still, they become frightened because of the consequences of what they might do wrong.

So, family, friends and colleagues at work may ask a sufferer to do something and they don't want to do it. And they repeatedly put if off but no-one understands why. And the sufferer can't explain easily that it is just because of how they feel.

Trying to remember things, especially when a sufferer is under pressure because people are waiting for them to decide or just being around them and waiting for a response to what has just happened can be physically as well as mentally exhausting. And once they start to forget, it just seems to get worse. And the worse it gets then the more exhausting it becomes.

Only where a sufferer can get out of the situation; where their inability to remember or process information isn't putting them under pressure do they stand any chance of recovery.

And, because people are almost always the source of the problem, this means a sufferer **HAS** to get out of the way of people. That's a difficult thing to explain to family, friends and colleagues at work.

Family and friends of sufferers often feel that this is an area where they can be of most help but to the sufferer it can often make things feel much worse.

For example, family and friends will write things down for the sufferer in the form of a list which they create to help them remember. But while the family and friends will see this as a "carrot" to encourage the sufferer to do things, the sufferer is far more likely to see it as a "stick" with which to be "mentally beaten" when the family member or friend returns later to check if they have done the things on the list.

The sufferer is not likely to want to talk about it and yet the family member or friend will see it as an opportunity to talk about "the sufferers day". The sufferer sees that as just another problem to add to the ones they already have – a bit like having lead weights tied to their legs while they are in the water and trying not to "mentally drown".

People want to communicate with a sufferer or expect things of them, particularly when they aren't well. And that requires them to think or do things. **But they CAN'T!**

Summary.

- **Dimension 9** is "Stars" and is all about the sufferer knowing where they are and their memory. "Stars" relates to the feeling of Memory Loss and Confusion. It is the second of the Green feelings. Sufferers become very forgetful; which can be very difficult for them at work and very frustrating for their family and friends. Working with lists is essential but they may also miss something that they should have done with one of the things on the list just because it wasn't written down. But these lists have to be their own lists. **When family and friends write their lists or ask them to do things it can feel like they are adding lead weights to their legs while they are in the water so increasing their feeling of "drowning".**

12 - Dimension 10 – Sun

Green

- *This refers mostly to the feeling of Hope.*

Now, unlike the rain, a bit of sunshine always seems to do people some good. Not too much to "burn" your skin but just enough to make you feel warm and comfortable.

And using the sunshine in this analogy, it is sunshine that gives us a feeling of **Hope.** It is the third and final Green feeling.

Without hope we really can get depressed and in this "water based analogy" I use "Sun" (Dimension 10) and sunshine as the opposite of rain as the "antidote" to depression. "Sun" relates to and is a measure of the feeling how hopeless or hopeful the sufferer feels in spite of how depressed they are.

Even when everything is going wrong there can still be moments when you see a ray of hope. I can remember once, many years ago, travelling by car through the country to an appointment.

I can't remember why but I was feeling pretty depressed that day although, at the time, I didn't know I suffered with depression. I decided that what I needed was a "spiritual uplift" so I decided to stop in the village called "Hope" and visit their really lovely little Church which I had passed many times before. I can remember that it was a weekday during the summer. It was lunchtime and the weather was warm but the sky was very cloudy.

I can remember thinking to myself, "What better spiritual message of hope can I give myself than to spend some quiet time in the Church at the centre of a village called "Hope".

So, I parked my car in the Church car-park and walked up through the Churchyard along the path between the gravestones worn away by time to the door of the Church and placed my hand on the door-handle. It was locked! A sign above the handle said, "This Church is closed today". No reason and no apology. I was in shock! I thought, "Even God has locked me out!"

So, here I was looking for hope at a Church in a village called "Hope" and even that was denied me. As I turned away I can remember starting to **laugh** as I thought to myself "What **hope** have I possibly got if I can't find hope at a Church in, of all places, a village called Hope".

I started to walk back to my car when suddenly a powerful shaft of really warm sunshine hit me and I looked up into the sky, saw the Sun appearing from behind a dark cloud, and suddenly I felt better.

Maybe it was God telling me something?

But I got the message that you don't have to go to "Hope" to find hope. Wherever you are and however bad you feel, you can find a little sunshine or belief anywhere and that can be a very powerful weapon in your fight against depression. And sufferers feel that they do have to fight depression. And they fight it every day.

So, I use "Sun" and sunshine as Dimension 10 to describe our ability to still have some **hope** and **belief** inside us that we will get better even though times can be hard. For a sufferer, the ability to find some hope from wherever it comes and wherever they can find it can just take a bit of the edge off what might otherwise be a serious episode of depression. Often that can come from the time they spend with people they know.

Sufferers who are depressed may always feel a little like they are "mentally drowning". But sometimes they need something to help them believe that they won't **actually** "mentally drown" and things can or will get better. There has to be at least some ray of hope that things can get better.

So, "Sun" (Dimension 10) is a measure of our feeling of hopelessness and our acceptance that in spite of everything **we can still find hope** or that we are able to accept it **can** exist.

Sufferers may not feel much hope at any given point in time but "Sun" (Dimension 10) is a measure of how strongly they feel it is out there waiting to be found somewhere. If they are to stand any chance of getting better then they need to have an inner feeling of hope so they can "bounce back" when the opportunity arises.

Now the difficult thing for family and friends to understand here is that you can't **give** sufferers hope. They have to **find** it themselves. It is a kind of **inner** strength. If they don't have it then no-one else can give it to them. And if they are ever likely to feel better then they need to find some of that **"Hope"**.

Summary.

- **Dimension 10** is "Sun" and is all about an inner feeling of hope. You might also describe it as optimism. It helps to have a sense of humour too. "Sun" relates to and is a measure of the feeling how hopeless or hopeful a sufferer feels in spite of everything. It is the third, last and, perhaps, the most important of the Green feelings. Depressed people really do have problems with Hope. It often eludes them and this is an important measure of their ability to "bounce back" when the time is right. **But it is important to understand that hope has to come from within the sufferer because you can't give sufferers hope - they have to find it for themselves.**

13 - Some other things to think about – especially family and friends.

No Model or Framework can be exhaustive and the 10 Dimensions I use to represent "feelings" don't describe a number of other situations that I think it is important to cover. I find it interesting that the more I, and other sufferers whom I have consulted, think about it there isn't much that can't be "simplistically" explained about a sufferers behaviour by reference to and an understanding of how the 10 Dimensions (feelings) I have identified work and a sufferers reaction to them.

But the following is a list of additional things that I know sufferers find difficult to explain to family and friends. They represent a short list in alphabetic order of the subjects on which **we are all agreed.**

I have also added to this Second Edition of the book, and under the heading for each of the following topics the Dimensions (feelings) most affected by the particular topic.

Alcohol

Dimension 1 - Sea Wave   *Overall*
feeling of
depression

Dimension 5 – Temperature   *Despair*

Let me begin by **making it clear** that if you suffer with depression then Doctors and Psychiatrists will recommend that **you don't drink alcohol** because alcohol causes depression or can make your current level of depression worse. That is especially true if you are on anti-depressants.

Whatever you do if you are a sufferer, don't just decide for yourself if you are OK to drink alcohol. **Ask your Doctor or Psychiatrist and listen to what they say. Do what they tell you because your needs are unique to you and they typically know best.**

If your Doctor does allow you the freedom to choose but you can't do so in moderation then alcohol isn't for you. I, together with a number of people whom I know who suffer with depression, have been advised that we can drink alcohol - but all of us do so in moderation. Most days I don't drink because I don't want to. But if I meet up with friends I am more inclined to. It requires discipline and an attitude of mind which, in spite of everything, enables you to always be in control. If you can't promise your Doctor or yourself that, then **never** drink alcohol.

Anger

Dimension 8 - Rain   *Stress*

Dimension 5 - Temperature   *Despair*

If you were a depressed person and you felt people around you were throwing those "buckets of water" over you then you might well feel the need to do whatever it takes to make them stop. Some people are already known to be prone to fits of temper and will become angry with those around them. Their depression just seems to make their anger worse.

However, there are other people who are not known for **ever** losing their temper. When they are depressed they can show uncharacteristic signs of anger which comes as a big surprise to family and friends who know them well and do not associate the sufferer with that emotion.

In order to understand why they feel the way they do you have to think about how ill and desperate they must feel in order for them to behave in this way. Aggression may be the only way that some sufferers feel they can respond in their effort to "defend themselves", survive their experience and stay "mentally alive".

Obviously, anger does not help the family and friends who are only trying to help. And, for family and friends, it must be very difficult to cope with anger and aggression when they really don't understand what the sufferer is going through. There is rarely an excuse for anger but, hopefully, the analysis and Dimensions (feelings) described in this book will go some way to explain it.

Conversation

Dimension 3 - River Current	*Isolation and vulnerability*
Dimension 5 - Temperature	*Despair*
Dimension 9 - Stars	*Memory loss and confusion*

Because a sufferer can become forgetful, and may also have a tendency to disengage with others when they are feeling unwell with depression, there is a feeling among family and friends that to involve a sufferer in their conversation may be either a waste of time or not what the sufferer seems able to enjoy. Both may be true and accurate assessments by those who know them best. And this may also apply more to men than women based on the generally accepted view that women enjoy and respond to conversation more than men.

However, the difficulty for the sufferer comes when they do feel the need to get involved but so much has happened since they last did and which they now know nothing about that it becomes embarrassing to the sufferer and them. It adds to their feeling of isolation and rejection, destroys their confidence and increases their feeling of failure to be part of the wider world in which they live.

There is a need for family and friends to involve a sufferer in conversation wherever possible but in such a way that they "gently" check for understanding as they go on. It isn't enough for them just to make statements and assume the sufferer knows and understands. It is even less appropriate not to check with them and assume that they have picked things up along the way. It is even worse if, because the sufferer doesn't seem to understand, they "speak at" the sufferer as if they are stupid.

Conversation is not necessarily communication. Many conversations are very one sided. Facts and opinions can only be communicated when replies from the listener indicate to the talker (and others) that the person listening has fully understood what the talker is saying. A sufferer is often in the position of not wanting or feeling able to respond properly and this can lead to a breakdown in communication which adds significantly to the sufferers feeling of isolation, hopelessness and despair. And it adds to the frustration of family and friends.

But, the responsibility for overcoming this issue has to lie with the speaker or non-sufferer as the sufferer may not be able to work out what is being talked about at the time. And it isn't their fault that they can't. It's because they are unwell.

Disappointment

Dimension 1 - Sea Wave   *Overall feeling of depression*

Dimension 3 - Lake Shore   *Isolation and vulnerability*

Dimension 10 - Sun   *Hope*

For no obvious reason, it seems that sufferers don't find it easy to deal with disappointment. Perhaps it's because they are trying really hard to overcome all of the issues which depression gives them that disappointment adds to their feeling of isolation and hopelessness. Being "left out" can be "disappointing". But, hope is inclusive and is the one thing that can overcome disappointment but sufferers don't always have it.

Family and friends really need to work together to ensure that the sufferer is, as far as possible, shielded from unnecessary disappointments which can seriously affect their feelings of hope and their overall feeling of depression.

Fear

Dimension 2 - River Current   *Duty and responsibility*

Dimension 4 - Time   *Need for support*

Dimension 7 - Wind   *Confidence*

Again, for no obvious reason, there seems to be a greater feeling of fear in sufferers. It can build up quickly and they may feel a much greater sensitivity to it. Perhaps it is because fear may affect their current level of depression, particularly in Dimension 2 – The "River Current", where sufferers try to shield themselves from any situation which might increase the intensity of the feeling.

It may also have something to do with the constant nervousness and awareness of the possibility that someone might want to pour some "buckets of water on them". So, although they may not show it, there is a tendency for them to have a constant low level of fear which can grow very quickly in situations where change is a possibility. That is especially true where a sufferer may have to do something which might require some of their "super human" effort.

Goodbyes and leaving.

Dimension 3 - Lake Shore   *Isolation and vulnerability*

Dimension 4 - Time   *Need for support*

Dimension 9 - Stars   *Memory loss and confusion*

There is often an irrational level of concern in a sufferer that when they say goodbye to someone they know well or love that this may be the last time they see them. Not because of any suicidal feelings or even a feeling in the sufferer that they might suddenly die but that their mental ability could suddenly let them down to such an extent that, in future, the sufferer may never remember who the friend or relative is. Or that something may go wrong with the relationship because of something they did or didn't do. Or something they didn't understand. And the sufferer may feel it was their fault. And that can create a self imposed feeling of guilt which is far more powerful and difficult to deal with than any guilt imposed on them by someone else.

Contact and time spent with family and friends may be much more valued by a sufferer than you might think. Always assuming they are not having "buckets of water" thrown on them, sufferers may place a high value on any time they spend with family and friends not least because they are often the best source of comfort and relief from how they feel. That particularly applies to those relatives and friends whom they don't see often and whose company they especially value.

Guilt.

Dimension 3 - Lake Shore   *Isolation and vulnerability*

Dimension 6 - Pressure   *Motivation*

Now, sometimes the people closest to the sufferer will use "guilt" to make a sufferer do something that they either can't or don't want to do. And the more that the sufferer submits to this approach the worse they feel. And yet the person who is the source of this approach increasingly sees their method as being effective. They don't understand the effect it is having on the sufferer they know and might love.

Over time, the sufferer will be much less affected by guilt as a method to get them to do something because the effort required to achieve what is being asked of them is often too much or makes them feel unwell. So, increasingly, they do not respond to the guilt imposed upon them. This can cause resentment in the relative or friend of the sufferer who thinks they are being disregarded or even ignored.

But because the sufferer may not have the vocabulary or ability to explain how they feel or what the "imposed guilt" is doing to them, they just use The "Lake Shore" (Dimension 3) to rescue themselves and "drift away from the shore" and contact with people as their best method of defence and self protection. Even if a sufferer did try and explain what it is doing to them, because people don't understand depression they often choose to disregard it. Friends and family often put it down to the sufferer just being awkward or lazy.

Laziness

Dimension 6 - Pressure   *Motivation*

Dimension 9 - Stars   *Memory loss and confusion*

Because a sufferer doesn't necessarily do things which might be staring them in the face as needing to be done, or that others want them to do, that doesn't necessarily mean they are lazy. While whatever it was that needed to be done just sat there, the sufferer may have been quietly trying subconsciously to recover from how they feel and that can be a "full time job" even if they are sat down or "aimlessly" walking around.

Or they may still be suffering and not wanting or feeling able to do much else. Or they may be concentrating on planning or doing something they feel they can do while more important things still wait to be started. Or they may have just forgotten. Or maybe they have forgotten how to do it or are worried that they may start something they won't be able to complete. It can be a mixture of all of these reasons.

So, if there are things to be done and the understanding, energy and motivation within the sufferer to do anything is low, they may choose to do whatever they feel is easiest, most pleasurable or most useful to them. It may not be at the top of the list in the eyes of the relative, friend or their Manager where they work. It might not even be on the list at all. And so it might seem to them that the sufferer is deliberately avoiding doing what is most important.

However, it is important to understand that if a sufferer is doing something, whatever that might be but which is useful to someone even if it is only the sufferer, then that is good. It is better than doing nothing because the sufferer is achieving something. And, although it may not be apparent to anyone else, the sufferer might be using a lot of energy or motivation which they may not have much of at the time.

Learning new things.

Dimension 7 - Wind	*Confidence*
Dimension 9 - Stars	*Memory loss and confusion*

Because sufferers often struggle to remember things, or use their brains to process things in a logical way, they are not very keen to try or learn new things with which they may not already be familiar. Classic examples of this are new technology products which surround us in our daily lives and upon which we often depend. There is often a tendency in sufferers to shy away from such things even though they may have been a highly competent and enthusiastic user of similar products in earlier times.

This lack of willingness to try new things may be a source of considerable frustration to family and friends. At work it could be a source of serious concern. But if a sufferer really does have a problem then having to deal with new things can seriously affect and increase their level of depression. Overcoming this "fear" can be difficult and can lead to both mental and physical exhaustion as they try to overcome it.

Listening

Dimension 3 - Lake Shore	*Isolation and vulnerability*
Dimension 9 - Stars	*Memory loss and confusion*

Good listening requires a conscious effort and can be very tiring. A sufferer, depending on how well they feel, may not have any spare mental capacity or energy left to listen properly so a conversation may appear to have gone normally whereas the sufferer may not have fully understood all that has been discussed.

So, sufferers are not always good listeners. And if they can't listen they won't understand and are far less likely to remember. And their ability to listen may also be dependent on the level of noise in the background. Perhaps there are distractions that are going on around them. Multi-tasking isn't an option for a sufferer when they aren't well. Even dealing with one thing may be too much.

Loneliness.

Dimension 3 - Lake Shore   *Isolation and vulnerability*

Dimension 4 - Time   *Need for support*

Depression seems to create in sufferers a very strong feeling of loneliness. They feel distant and remote even from people who are nearby and with whom they are in a relationship. But occasionally they tend to over-compensate for this feeling. While sometimes they feel the need to get out of the way of other people, at other times they feel the urgent need to have company. There is even a tendency for them to want to stay with others when the others are busy and have things to do and get on with. They seem to have an unreasonable desire to get family and friends to stay when they need to go. They sometimes seem frightened to be left alone.

One of the things which makes it more difficult for sufferers to "swim away from the shore" to get some peace is that they don't want to go too far in case they do feel lonely and vulnerable. So, they have to strike a balance between getting the peace of mind they need and increasing their feelings of isolation and loneliness.

They don't always get it right and when they get it wrong that can make them feel much worse particularly if they feel they may have offended family and friends in the process. Family and friends need to take this issue into account during their daily and ongoing contact with the sufferer they know.

Noise

Dimension 2 - River Current   *Duty and responsibility*

Dimension 7 - Wind   *Confidence*

Sufferers do not seem to like sudden or sustained loud noises.

Loud noise **demands** immediate attention and change. It interrupts whatever other sounds are around which might include conversation, music or some other sound which a sufferer is trying to listen to. Because a sufferer may already be desperately trying to stay involved and understand whatever other sounds they are listening to, loud noise can seriously affect the level of their feelings in one or more of the Dimensions.

It particularly affects the "River Current" (Dimension 2) and sudden or sustained loud noise can suddenly and dramatically increase the level in that Dimension from between 10 and 20 (level 2) to as much as 80 to 90 (level 9). That can be unbearable not least because it is a sudden and immediate change. It really does feel as if you have been suddenly thrown into a raging fast flowing "mental river" and that you are, "mentally", being violently swept away at great speed. It can be a cause of an angry response.

So, it isn't the impact on the ear that is so serious, even though that may be bad enough, it is what it is doing to the brain and how the brain tries to cope with it. Moreover, whereas the ear might recover in a short time, it might take the sufferer some time to recover mentally. Sufferers may feel the need to go somewhere quiet to overcome the effect. They may seek the safety of a significant distance from the "Lake Shore" to get away from the source of the noise.

Obsession

Dimension 9 - Stars   *Memory   loss and confusion*

Sufferers often behave in an obsessive way about things. That may be partly due to the fact that they like things to be done properly so, where others around them may have partly finished something and moved on, they stick with it to ensure it is properly finished long after others have any interest.

Possibly another of the reasons why sufferers behave in an obsessive way is that they have a need to focus on something which works for them and that they have confidence in. Or that they feel the need to work harder and for longer to make sure they are happy that what they are doing is correct. Or maybe during the process their concentration is affected and they have to focus harder and longer to get it right. As part of the forgetfulness that comes with depression, they may fear that they have missed something.

Equally, sufferers have difficulty dealing with more than one thing at a time when they are ill. So there may well be a tendency to over-compensate by being seemingly "obsessed" with what they feel they are competent to do without realising how that appears to others. Staying within their comfort zone seems narrow and obsessive to others who may be multi-tasking or managing several things where the sufferer is only dealing with one.

Sleep

Dimension 1 - Sea Wave   *Overall feeling of depression*

Dimension 6 - Pressure   *Motivation*

When sufferers are depressed there is a tendency for them to sleep longer. Where previously 8 hours would do and they could wake up refreshed, maybe they suddenly need 10 hours. Sometimes, even 12 hours may not be enough. And when they wake up, they might still feel exhausted.

Depression has the effect of tiring you out in a way that sleep alone doesn't help resolve. Yes, it is much better if you are in a routine and early nights are beneficial.

There are two "sayings" I know of about sleep:-

- "Early to bed and early to rise, makes a man healthy, wealthy and wise".

- "An hour of sleep before midnight is worth two hours after midnight".

I don't believe the bit about wealthy but I do believe the rest about health and wisdom. And I also believe in the benefit of getting to bed before midnight. You know that if you are tired your brain doesn't work as well? Which is why, if depression makes you tired anyway, you can get into a descending cycle of worsening health if you aren't careful.

So, if a sufferer is unwell then getting to bed at a sensible time (say between 10:00 and 10:30 p.m.) each night is a really good idea. But it is equally important to have to get up at a sensible time. If they don't naturally wake up by 7:00 or 8:00 a.m. then they need to set an alarm.

There will be many mornings when the "Sea Wave" (Dimension 1) may be quite big, either when they wake up naturally or the alarm goes off, but it doesn't help to just stay in bed. Even if they don't go out or do anything special, it is good to get up and take a shower or bath if they normally do and, **most importantly,** get dressed. After that, they should have a breakfast of whatever they normally enjoy. It may not make a big difference but it is a positive routine and it helps.

Success versus Survival.

Dimension 2 - River Current   *Duty and responsibility*

Dimension 6 - Pressure   *Motivation*

I have already said that I believe, and history points out many excellent examples, that depressed people are often very clever and successful, and high achievers too. They typically achieve success between bouts of depression. But, they can still achieve great things even during a depressive episode although that can be extremely exhausting for them, both physically and mentally. Many argue that artists who suffer with depression achieve their best work when they are in the deepest of their depressions.

In the Family and Friends Guide in Appendix 2 at the end of the book, in the lower levels I have identified, say between 10 and 30, then a sufferer is at their best and will want to achieve all that they can. At this level (levels 1 to 3) sufferers are highly motivated by **Success**.

Remember that I have already explained that on the scale I have used you **can't** have a score lower than 10 because the lowest score in each of the 10 Dimensions is 1. So if you add them all up it will add up to a minimum of 10.

At the other end of the scale, say between 70 and 90 (remember that between 90 and 100 sufferers are unlikely to be able to do anything) they are only interested in being able to survive whatever is being asked of them or whatever it is that they are trying to achieve for themselves. So at the top end of the scale (levels 8 to 10) their main, or perhaps only, motivation is **Survival.**

So, in between 30 and 70 (levels 4 to 7) sufferers find themselves sitting between the extremes and having progressively mixed feelings of Motivation towards Success or Survival depending upon how they feel at the time. As a result, their decision-making process may be affected.

I can remember one friend who suffers with depression saying "I never make any decisions when I feel depressed because they are almost always bad decisions". At the time I felt I understood what they were saying because it was sensible for them not to do anything at such a time. However, now that I understand about the levels of feeling, and the different levels of Motivation for Success or Survival, for the first time I really feel that I do actually **know what they mean.**

Tasks

Dimension 2 - River Current	*Duty and responsibility*
Dimension 6 - Pressure	*Motivation*
Dimension 7 - Wind	*Confidence*

Family and friends often feel that the best way to help a sufferer is to involve them in what they are doing or to give them something to do while they are away. **Nothing could be further from the truth.**

A sufferer often struggles to deal with a few things they have to do or have decided to do themselves. Being asked to do more or change what they have already started or planned can seriously and adversely affect how they feel. If a sufferer feels well they will be able to Multi-task and do a wide range of things just like anyone else. But as they progressively feel worse, their ability to do more than one thing at the same time decreases until, when they are really ill, they can't even do one thing.

A depressed person is usually trying as best as they can to deal with what they absolutely **have** to do. If they **don't** have to do anything then they tend to use this time to find that calm stretch of "water" so they can mentally rest. Don't forget, coping with depression is a full time "job".

So, involving sufferers in things they may not feel up to, or even don't want to do, can only make things worse. Sometimes very much worse and often, because the sufferer doesn't want to hurt the feelings of the relative or friend whom they know is only trying to help, they allow themselves to be "dragged along" even though inside their head they know it is making them feel worse.

When family and friends "give a sufferer something to do" they have no idea what it can be like to be on the receiving end.

On a good day, asking a sufferer to do something may be just the same as asking someone who isn't a sufferer and the effort involved may be minor. However, later the same day that could change for the sufferer but the person who gave you the task only remembers how you were at the time. No-one knows how the day might progress, least of all the sufferer. On another day when they feel ill, it can be awful.

On a bad day, asking a sufferer to do something simple can be as unrealistic as asking them to climb Everest (the highest mountain in the world) alone and without help in the dark. The sufferer might look OK to you so you wouldn't think twice about asking. And because the sufferer might not want to hurt your feelings, they may go through a "living hell" to try and do it and, afterwards, will be both mentally and physically exhausted. You may come back and find the sufferer asleep in a chair and you might wonder what all the fuss is about. But to the sufferer, they may be just pleased to have mentally survived the experience.

So, tasks and delegation are a problem for sufferers. It all goes back to duty and responsibility. Sometimes they are up to it and other times they aren't. But it isn't their fault when they aren't because they may not be well enough to do it.

Telephone Calls

| *Dimension 2 - River Current* | *Duty and responsibility* |
| *Dimension 6 - Pressure* | *Motivation* |

People telephone others for a variety of reasons. But mostly they require a level of involvement by the receiver to listen to them and respond appropriately. That requires concentration and the ability to hear and understand.

Depending on how ill they feel, a sufferer may not want to answer the telephone even when it is a relative or friend calling to see how they are simply because they may not be able to deal with all that the call might involve. And they may also not feel able to **make** a telephone call for the same reason.

Bear in mind that their ability may also be affected by noise and volume and the need to take on new information which has to be understood or perhaps remembered. All of these are potential factors that can affect how depressed a sufferer becomes. It mainly affects the "River Current" (Dimension 2).

Tiredness

Dimension 2 - River Current   *Duty and responsibility*

Dimension 6 - Pressure   *Motivation*

Most people think that Sleep and Tiredness are connected. Well, for a sufferer, the connection is not as clear as you might think.

Depression seems to make your brain work far harder than it should normally have to. Because it all seems to be happening in their subconscious it can appear to others that a sufferer is just sat there doing nothing, while they feel increasingly tired as they do. If they have to do something that they hadn't planned to which causes their "River Current" (Dimension 2) to increase dramatically then they may find that they are mentally and physically exhausted in a very short time.

So, if the sufferer is constantly yawning, it isn't necessarily just because they are bored or physically tired or even because they haven't slept well. It could be because they are going through a depressive episode and are in the phase where their brain is either coping or "calming down" and the "waves" are slowly subsiding.

It can be both annoying and puzzling to family and friends if a sufferer can't stop yawning when it appears to them that they haven't done anything. If you can remember the example I gave earlier where I only made a cup of coffee, I was both physically and mentally exhausted afterwards and I couldn't stop yawning till I went to bed.

Waking up.

Dimension 1 - Sea Wave	*Overall feeling of depression*
Dimension 2 - Lake Shore	*Duty and responsibility*
Dimension 4 - Time	*Need for support*

It is important to understand that when a sufferer wakes up they are likely to feel at least one and maybe two (or more) levels worse than they will in a few hours time. That is always assuming nothing happens to make them feel worse. This "morning feeling" is well documented by those who are medically qualified.

For example, using the scale shown in the Family and Friends Guide in Appendix 2 at the end of the book, if a sufferer normally feels between 30 and 40 (level 4) then it is likely that they may wake up feeling at least between 40 and 50 (level 5). They might even feel as bad as between 80 and 90 (level 9). So, the first few hours of each day can often be tough. But by lunchtime they may feel much better.

So, not only does a sufferer have to cope with whatever the new day is presenting, they also start at a disadvantage. Sometimes that can be a big disadvantage. And no-one but the sufferer knows how ill they really feel. It can require a huge amount of effort to work their way through this period until they feel better. And, ironically, they can become increasingly exhausted as they do.

Summary

From what you have read in this **Chapter 13 – "Some other things to think about - especially family and friends"** you can see that there are a lot of external factors from such diverse topics as "tasks" and "noise", which can seriously affect how sufferers feel. It can be hard for family and friends who don't suffer with depression to understand why sufferers are affected in the way they are and these factors don't easily fit into any of the "Dimensions".

Having discussed the above issues (and many more besides) with a significant number of sufferers, these additional factors that I have included in his Chapter do seem to affect most if not all sufferers and their depression so it is important for sufferers and their family and friends to understand these things and take them into account.

Wherever a consensus of opinion can be achieved on any other topics, I will include them in any later version of this book.

14 - Some things that seem to help - and some others that don't.

The following few suggestions are made as a guide to how you might support a relative or friend who suffers with depression. These are not rigid and not taken from any "clinically approved list".

But they are based on conversations and discussions I have had with other sufferers and non-sufferers and they represent some of the things that they and I feel most helpful or which makes them feel worse.

I've divided them into two lists of 10 things which I show on the following pages.

Firstly - Some things to remember which sufferers seem to find helpful.

1   Always remember that depression is not a "visible illness". Depression is hidden. You can't easily see when or the degree to which a sufferer is either well or ill not least because they may be hiding it from you. You can't know what is going on and sometimes, neither does the sufferer. So, suggesting or insisting that a sufferer does something at any point in time may not be helpful and could make them feel much worse. For no obvious reason or visible change, in a short while they may feel quite different. So, when necessary, it is important and most helpful to gauge and work with the sufferer to establish how they feel and not try to force the pace.

2   Always try and be supportive. Sufferers need it even though, from the feedback they give you, it may seem to you as if they don't want it and don't care.

3   It is important to always try and be positive. Negativity, criticism and not being helpful really can feel to a sufferer very much like having "buckets of water" thrown over

them. I feel sure that **you** wouldn't throw water on a drowning man. So **why** "metaphorically" do it to someone you know or love.

4   If it is normal for the sufferer to be open with you then do take time to find out how they feel and take it into account in how you deal with them.

5   As far as possible, do let the sufferer dictate the pace. They may be going as fast as they mentally and physically can. Don't forget, depression causes both serious mental and physical tiredness.

6   Wherever possible spend time with your relative or friend if they want to but leave them if they don't. Enjoy with them the days that they are well. Sometimes it is the memory of the good days that make the difference for a sufferer in getting through a bad day.

7   It is important to always remember that a sufferer would desperately love for their depression to end and there are days when they are quietly suffering in a way that, for them, can be almost too awful for you to imagine.

8 When you are with someone who is a sufferer look for the signs that they may not be coping and are unwell. They may not be able to see it themselves. Sometimes they need help before they realise it.

9 Try and understand all of the Dimensions and the "other things" in "Chapter 13 – some other things to think about - especially family and friends" that can affect how a sufferer feels and what they feel able to do as a result.

10 And always remember that they will have some level of depression - even on a day when they seem completely well. For them coping with depression is a full time "job".

Second – some things that DON'T seem helpful to them.

1   Don't blame sufferers for being depressed. Sometimes they can't do anything about it more than they are already trying to do every day of their lives. You may never understand how hard they have to try some days. They would just love to be able to "get out of the water and get dry", just like you are every day of your life.

2   It is most unhelpful to create unnecessary situations or problems for the sufferer. It can make an already difficult day seem almost impossible to get through. So, try not to "throw buckets of water" on your already drowning relative or friend!

3   It is important not to dismiss or reject them, or create barriers which affect the day to day relationships on which they may significantly rely even though you may not realise it because they don't show it or admit it. Sufferers are vulnerable most of the time and feel it very deeply when things affect them.

4 Don't force them to be with people at times when they need to be on their own. Within reason, let them choose the kind of "therapy" and people to be with which best suits their needs at the time. It is also important not to misunderstand their reasons if they choose friends over family during difficult times.

5 Showing your annoyance when they are having a bad day makes them feel worse and some sufferers aren't able mentally to defend themselves at times from the awful effects of conflict or rejection.

6 Sufferers may, at times, feel unable to do things which you need or want them to do. So, it is most unhelpful to try and force them to do things or even to try and force them **NOT** to do something which might be reasonable for them to want to do.

7 Don't force any changes on the situation of a sufferer or persuade them to take risks if they don't want to. You may not see something as "a risk" but the risk might seem to them to be far too great.

8 Adding to the difficulties they may already feel they are submerged under is especially unhelpful. Try where possible to understand their needs and offer help if there is anything they will let you do to help them.

9   Don't give a sufferer tasks to do in the belief it will keep them "occupied" and take things "off their mind". Depression seems mostly to do with what is happening in the subconscious so what they "consciously" do may have little or no positive effect. But it could easily make them feel much worse. Lists seem to be a special issue. If they want help with theirs that is fine. But they have to write their own. It has to be theirs.

10   Perhaps most important of all try not to do or say anything that denies them hope of achieving what they set out to do. Hope is one of the most precious things they have "inside" and it is often difficult to regain it if lost.

15 - Some Final Words

At the beginning of the book I explained that I am not a qualified person in any form of Mental Health but the feedback I have received from the sufferers and non-sufferers I have had discussions with lead me to believe that what I have written can be and has already been of help. Perhaps it might help you or someone you know and love!

In fact, all of the people who read the first drafts and First Edition, whether they were a sufferer or a non-sufferer, told me that it helped them in some way or another.

So, in writing the book in the way I have, I have tried to create something which is practical and I aimed it at two distinct groups of people to be used every day:-

- Partly those who are suffering with depression in the hope they may learn something about themselves through my experience and analysis that will help them better communicate with those around them and thereby help them cope and perhaps even improve their daily lives.

- But **MOSTLY** at those who do **NOT** suffer with depression but who hope to learn something about how it feels so that they can talk to and help a relative or friend and in so doing make everyones' lives that little bit better.

When discussing depression with other sufferers I did agree with them that my own experience with depression may well be very different to everyone else who suffers with it. And that the way I have described it may not be the same for everyone else either.

But most of the reviewers, including Doctors and Psychiatrists, agreed that the way I use the metaphors for the feelings (such as the "Wind" and "Rain") did provide a useful tool for family and friends to talk to the sufferer; in order to get a better understanding of how it feels to the sufferer they know and love. And that might enable them to get a better understanding of how to help them.

As I have already mentioned in Chapter 1 – Introduction, one of sufferers I have known for many years once said to me, "You can't deal with depression all at once. You have to deal with it bit by bit". One of the main reasons why people say they like this book is that it explains the different feelings in "bite sized pieces".

Perhaps the most useful thing about the 10 Dimensions (feelings) I have identified and which works for me is that at any time I can assess numerically exactly how I feel in each of the Dimensions (feelings) and, when I have to, I can focus on what helps me feel better in each one. Or, most importantly, I can deal with the one which I know is worst and when I feel better in that one I am more able to deal with the others.

So, the message for sufferers is that if, by talking to family and friends they know how you are feeling and which of the feelings is worst for you at any point in time, they can be of much more help because no-one is guessing about how you feel any more.

Family and friends can help you focus on the exact thing that is best for you. But, most importantly, if you are the sufferer now you can understand too which may leave you in better control of your improvements. If everyone works together life gets better for everybody.

Let me finish with a few words for each of these two groups of people I have aimed the book at, starting with those who sufferer with depression.

Note to the Sufferers

I hope that you got some benefit out of the book and, if it has helped you even in the slightest way, then I am pleased. Following the First Edition I have had some excellent and moving feed-back as to how people have identified with the way I have described depression. Perhaps you have other experiences of other Dimensions that I haven't even thought about.

I especially hope it has helped you in one or both of the following 2 ways:-

- To be able to analyse for yourself how you feel at any point in time and thereby enable you to work out ways in which to help yourself feel better and prevent yourself from feeling worse.

- To be able to talk about how you feel with family and friends so that you can work together to improve how you feel and how your feelings impact those around you.

I wish you a pleasant journey through the rest of your life and I express the hope that in your lifetime, if not mine, somebody finds a "real" cure so that we, the sufferers, can party together on that elusive patch of "dry land" maybe on a beach somewhere.

But, trust me, if I ever get out of the "water" and get "dry", I will not be going back in the "water". **Ever!**

Note to the Family and Friends

I hope you have learned something from the book. In particular I hope you have learned 3 things:-

- That it is a serious and extremely unpleasant condition for the sufferer about which there is still much to be learned. I am sure that you are glad you don't suffer with it?

- That your relative or friend who suffers with depression needs a lot of help from time to time. And although it may seem like they don't appreciate your help and understanding, they do but can't always respond in a way that would make sense to you or them. But talking to them may be of real help to them.

- To be there for them at "the beach party" and to celebrate with them when hopefully, in time and with new treatments, they finally "come ashore and get dry".

Finally

In the First Edition of this book I based what I wrote primarily on my own experience but influenced by what I learned from other sufferers, family and friends and the three original Doctors who helped me with advice as I wrote it.

In this Second Edition of the book I have made some changes based on the comments and advice I have been given by hundreds of people who were either sufferers or their family and friends.

I have especially listened to the many additional Doctors and Psychiatrists who were kind enough to give me the benefit of their expert feedback.

So, this book should be **MUCH** more relevant than ever for sufferers and their family and friends in developing a better mutual understanding of what it is like to suffer with depression and how to deal with it in a mutually helpful way.

Hopefully people will continue to find this book to be of practical help for sufferers with depression, their family and friends because of the way it helps people discuss depression and thereby make a positive difference to so many peoples' lives.

If you want to be made aware of any developments after the publication of this Second Edition, **please refer to my blog site** - note that it ends in **"ORG"**

<u>www.thealreadydrowningman.org</u>

THE END

Appendices

Appendices

Appendix 1 – Self Assessment

The Self Assessment Chart

This chart is a Self Assessment Chart to help the sufferer get an idea of how they feel at a particular time. Only the sufferer can complete it because only they know how they feel. Each of the points refers to a different Dimension (feeling) numbered 1 to 10. Each of the Dimensions has a scale of intensity from 1 to 10 where 1 is where you feel really good and 10 is a measure of how bad you really feel when at its' worst.

You have to put in the box for each row the number that most accurately reflects how you feel and you have to do all 10 of the Dimensions at the same time as you may have a different mix of feelings in an hour. It you aren't sure what one of the Questions means then go back to the Chapter which covers that Dimension and read the prompt at the end.

It may help you to keep a record of how you feel so we have added below some boxes to put in the relevant data for the day of the week, date, location and time of day.

- Day of the week
- Date
- Location
- Time of day

Dimen-sion	Note that when entering your scores you can only enter a score of 1 up to 10.	Enter your score in the boxes below
1	Overall, just how depressed do you feel now? How big are the waves?	
2	How badly are the day to day demands getting on top of you right now? How anxious do you feel?	
3	How vulnerable or isolated do you feel right now? How far are you from the shore?	
4	How bad is the need for or the benefit you get from support making you feel now?	

5	How serious is the current level of your feeling of despair?	
6	How deep is the level to which you feel totally de-motivated?	
7	How comfortable are you with the current level of your fear of risk and change? How confident are you?	
8	How great are the level of difficulties you feel that you currently have to cope with in your life? How stressed do you feel?	
9	How badly are you affected by the inability of your brain to remember things or work things out? How forgetful or confused are you?	
10	How deep is the level of hopelessness you feel?	

What is your total score?

Add up all of the numbers as you have scored them. A low score is good and a high score is bad. Out of 100 today, how do you feel? How does that compare with your most common score? Do you know what your most common score is?	

Describe in only 1 word how you feel right now.	

Now you know how you feel in each of the 10 Dimensions above. You may have replaced some of my Dimensions (feelings) with others of your own which is fine.

Remember, in order to try and improve the way you feel it is important to try and deal first with the feeling which has the highest score. You need to work out what helps you feel better for each of the 10 Dimensions. There won't just be one thing - there could easily be a few. Write them down so you don't forget them because on some days you may not be able to remember any of them or be able to do your first choice.

Why not use the blank form in Appendix 4 – "Things that can help you" to record them as you work out what helps you and what doesn't for each of the feelings or what I have called Dimensions.

Also, don't just do what makes you feel better in one Dimension without thinking about what it does for the others. You need to work out what is the best combination of things that helps you on the day.

Appendix 2 – Family and Friends Guide

The Family and Friends' Guide to the interpretation of the Self Assessment Chart

Scores.

In order to get some measure of how unwell a sufferer with depression might feel and how their responsiveness to involvement and support might work, the following is a "**very rough guide**". Remember, this is not a "clinically recognised" method.

At the risk of confusing you here, I have chosen to use the Red, Amber and Green method of analysis (I have also used them to classify the different Dimensions) in order to help prioritise the different levels of how a sufferer feels.

Clearly, a sufferers need for support and how you might deal with them will need to vary according to whether they feel they are in the "Green", "Amber" or "Red" Zone. Anyone in the Red zone for more than a short time should see a Doctor urgently. Any sufferer who is regularly in the Amber zone needs to be under the care of a Doctor too.

People tend to assume that only in the worst cases (above 80%) should they really need to take any notice of how a sufferer feels. But, the important thing to note is that, on this scale, **sufferers with scores of as low as 50% may find difficulty in doing things.** Even with scores as low as 60%, sufferers are already quite unwell but may still be hiding it and trying to put on a brave face so as not to "let everyone down". By 70% their ability to do things is seriously affected and by 80% they are already really ill!

So, it is important to be ready to offer support at 50% and not assume they are OK until they reach 80%.

Another thing to remember is that the changes in level, especially increases, can happen quickly and be as much as 30% in either direction. In extreme circumstances the change can be as high as 40% or more. So a sufferer can easily go from 30% to 70% or even higher while still in your company.

They may have felt fine at first and may not understand why things have changed. And you may not even notice until well into the change. It is important to understand that change is far more likely than not so don't assume that the level your relative or friend started with will be the same when you or they leave.

Score	Red, Amber or Green	General feeling	Ability to respond to involvement and support
Level 1 **0 - 10**		**Exceptional.** This is actually a totally unrealistic score. If you add up each Dimension with a minimum score of 1, then the minimum you will get is 10. You can't have 9 or less.	**Exceptional.** Perfectly normal behaviour and competence. No tiredness and memory is excellent.
Level 2 **10 – 20**	**Green 1**	**Excellent.** Probably as good as a sufferer with depression is ever likely to feel	**Excellent.** Will still seem perfectly normal and will act normal. Will probably be able to withstand anything that can happen. Again, no tiredness and memory is excellent.

Level 3 20 - 30	Green 2	Very Good. Sufferers would like to feel like this most days.	Very Good. Will join in on 99% of all things. Will feel able to achieve most things and even if you know them well you would not recognise anything abnormal in them. No obvious tiredness and memory is good
Level 4 30 - 40	Green 3	Good. Perhaps the average sort of day.	Good. This is the first level at which the sufferer becomes aware that they are not well. There may be a hesitance to get involved in or do things. There may be a tendency to put things off if they don't need to be done urgently. Occasional slight tiredness and memory may need prompting.

Level 5 40 – 50	Amber 1	OK on some days. Depending on the mix of feelings, this might be a more difficult day	Average. At this level the sufferer is definitely aware that they are not 100% but is sufficiently motivated to try and overcome the way they feel. They may not want to try and do something that they don't have to do or upon which they may be judged. Tiredness may become more obvious and memory may be suspect. Ability to remember how to do things also slightly affected.
Level 6 50 – 60	Amber 2	Not so good. Again, depending on the mix of feelings on any day, this day could be really a	Below average. When the sufferer is at this level everything becomes an effort. Keeping themselves motivated is

		bit of a struggle for a sufferer. They may look and act distracted.	difficult and they will begin to feel tired for no obvious reason. They will yawn and may sit down at every opportunity. They will make an effort when called upon but only for short periods. Memory is clearly affected and so is the ability to remember how to do things.
Level 7 **60 – 70**	**Amber** **3**	**Quite unwell.** May have difficulty in attempting some things which most people would regard as normal. For those that know what to look for, you will be able to see and detect this level clearly.	**Poor.** This is the highest level at which the sufferer will feel any normal motivation to do anything. They will involve themselves but may not feel able to complete things normally. Their staying power is low. They are beginning to feel uncontrollably tired. Even sitting

			down doesn't help. Their willingness to do things or get involved is very much at the lowest end of the scale. Memory can often be poor. Ability to do things is clearly affected by an inability to remember how.
Level 8 70–80	Red 1	Feeling quite ill. Would definitely seem unable to do a wide range of things. Unlikely to respond to most normal external attempts at support. This is the first level at which their general lack of well being is easily seen even by those that don't know what to look for.	Very poor. This is the first level at which they have real difficulty in doing almost anything. They don't want to get involved and certainly won't welcome any tasks being assigned to them. Expecting anything to be done when the sufferer is at this level is unrealistic. But they can and will do things where the need is

			great. They are almost always very tired and although they may at times make an effort, they will quickly tire and give up. Remembering anything is an effort as is the ability to remember how to do things. They need to know they have support and have things done for them.
Level 9 **80 - 90**	**Red** **2**	**Very ill.** Unwilling or unable to participate in almost anything. They appear and act very tired and exhausted both in their looks and demeanour. May cause concern in people who are	**Difficult.** This is a very difficult level for the sufferer. They are very Depressed and have a strong feeling of despair. They do not want to do anything and it would be unwise to involve them in anything. Only super human effort will get them through this and

		nearby and don't know the sufferer.	let them achieve anything. They need support even though they may not want it or recognise it. They can hardly remember anything and do not remember how to do many things. They do need lots of things done for them. They need medical care. Achieving anything requires super human effort.
Level 10 **90 -** **100**	**Red** **3**	**Seriously ill.** There will be absolutely no doubt in your mind that the sufferer you know is seriously ill. They may not get out of bed but once up they will struggle to	**Impossible.** Totally unresponsive. Impossible to get sufferers view on how they feel so scores of this high may never be obtained from them directly but can only be guessed at. Not able or willing to do anything or even try. They are

		move around. Normal daily hygiene routines will be absent. At this level, they may be a danger to themselves or others. Those that don't know the sufferer well might feel the need to call an ambulance or a Doctor.	really beyond even the "super human" effort stage. Absolutely exhausted mentally, physically, emotionally and spiritually. They may not even remember family or friends. They don't remember how to do most things even the simplest of tasks. They need medical care more than anything. Support is still important for them but they are unlikely to recognise it, respond to it or show any appreciation for it.

Appendix 3 – The Summaries

Bullet Point Summary

The following list is a collection of all of the bullet points at the end of each of the 10 Dimensions assembled in one place for you to look at and to help you remember them. But we start with the three main ones which underpin everything.

From Chapter 1 - the most important bullet points are these.

- If you **DON'T** suffer with depression then, in this analogy, you are **ALWAYS** on land or on the ship and you are always "**DRY**".

- If you **DO** suffer from depression then, in this analogy, **you are ALWAYS in the water. You NEVER get out of the water and you are always "WET".**

- Depression is a **complex mixture of feelings** each of which can be described as a different "Dimension" (feeling). You will always score at least 1 out of 10 in each them, even on a good day. On good days you can feel 2 out of 10 in some of them but on days when you feel ill you could feel over 7 out of 10 in most of them.

Now for the Dimensions in Chapters 3 to 12.

- **Dimension 1** is the "Sea Wave" and is the main Dimension. It is the first and most important of the Red feelings. This relates to the overall feeling of Depression and is perhaps both the cause and the consequence of all of the others. It is the one over which a sufferer has no control. It's the way their brain is working when they wake up and nothing they can do during the day will necessarily make it better. **It may get better on its' own but, typically, the other Dimensions can only make it worse.**

- **Dimension 2** is the "River Current" and the next most serious feeling. It is the second Red feeling. I believe it is the "River Current" which most relates to the feelings of Anxiety. And it is the feeling which many people associate with Panic Attacks. It is the one which reflects a sufferers' daily life and, because it is the one which they can sometimes do something about, it can often be the reason why they hide away. **Adding to the sufferers' problems is like throwing bucket loads of water on an already drowning man.**

- **Dimension 3** is the "Lake Shore" and is a measure of how good the support is or how sufferers benefit from the help their family and friends, and Professionals including Counsellors give them. The "Lake Shore" refers to the feelings of Isolation and Vulnerability. It is the third and final Red feeling. The distance from the "Lake Shore" is a measure of how isolated or vulnerable they feel and, subject to the quality of the support, they will either swim towards the shore or away from it. Family and friends need to understand how to get the sufferer to "swim towards them". They also need to understand that whatever they do and however hard they try to help, the sufferer just may not be able to swim any closer. **And, to the sufferer, all the love in the world may not be enough to help them at that time.**

- **Dimension 4** is "Time". "Time" relates to the feelings of "Need for" or the "Benefit of Support". It is the first of the Amber (Yellow) feelings. It can refer to the time they have suffered with depression or even how long a depressive episode can last. But mostly it refers to the time sufferers spend with people and how family, friends and work colleagues can have a widely differing effect on helping them feel better. Even the closest family member may not be the best person to help. Sometimes, duty and responsibility towards family makes it more difficult. **The best help comes from people a sufferer chooses to be with.**

- **Dimension 5** is "Temperature". So "Temperature" relates to the level of a sufferers' feeling of Despair. It is the second but perhaps most important of the Amber (Yellow) feelings. It is a broad measure of despair and the lower the temperature then the deeper is the despair. While a sufferer can try and lift themselves out of this feeling sometimes it just isn't possible. And while family, friends and colleagues at work may try to help, at the end of the day, only they can achieve it. **And much to the annoyance of those around the sufferer, on some days they neither can nor want to.**

- **Dimension 6** is "Pressure" and is all about the feeling of Motivation (the inner pressure to do something). It is the third of the Amber (Yellow) feelings. Depression affects a sufferers' motivation. And if a sufferer has to motivate themselves to do even the simplest of tasks it can be absolutely exhausting. Expecting someone with depression to do things may not be realistic. It isn't that they are lazy but at times they lack the Motivation to do things that anyone else might do easily and without effort. Lack of purpose will make things worse. **Forcing sufferers to do things that they see no point in or don't feel able to do because of low Motivation can make their depression worse to the extent that they then increase the distance from the "Lake Shore" (Dimension 3) by swimming away from safety and support.**

- **Dimension 7** is "Wind" and is all about Change. "Wind" relates to the feelings associated with change and a sufferers' ability to deal with it because of their level of Confidence. It is the fourth and last of the Amber (Yellow) feelings. People who are depressed do not like change and have perhaps a higher than normal resistance to it. It is important to get some idea of a sufferers ability to cope with change as that can have a big affect on how they deal with it, and how that affects the other Dimensions, when change comes their way. Equally, sufferers avoid risk, even though they might not seem to care anymore. **Although sufferers might desperately want change for the better they fear change because for them it always seems to get worse or can make them feel ill.**

- **Dimension 8** is "Rain" and is all about what is going on or wrong in a sufferers life. It may even be a measure of the subconscious issues that they have. "Rain" relates to the feeling of Stress. It is the first of the Green feelings. Is life difficult? If it is, then Dimension 8 is the place where a sufferer can take account of that feeling. And it is important to understand whether or not things are going well because it makes everything else so difficult if they are trying to cope and want to benefit from support. **When things around a sufferer are difficult it is a bit like being anchored miles (kilometres) from the "Lake Shore" and out of reach of the help they want and need.**

- **Dimension 9** is "Stars" and is all about the sufferer knowing where they are and their memory. "Stars" relates to the feeling of Memory Loss and Confusion. It is the second of the Green feelings. Sufferers become very forgetful which can be very difficult for them at work and very frustrating for their family and friends. Working with lists is essential but they may also miss something that they should have done with one of the things on the list just because it wasn't written down. But these lists have to be their own lists. When family and friends write their lists or ask them to do things it can feel like they are adding lead weights to their legs while they are in the water so increasing their feeling of "drowning".

- **Dimension 10** is "Sun" and is all about an inner feeling of Hope. You might also describe it as optimism. It helps to have a sense of humour too. "Sun" relates to and is a measure of the feeling how hopeless or hopeful a sufferer feels in spite of everything. It is the third, last and, perhaps, the most important of the Green feelings. Depressed people really do have problems with Hope. It often eludes them and this is an important measure of their ability to "bounce back" when the time is right. **But it is important to understand that hope has to come from within the sufferer because you can't give sufferers hope - they have to find it for themselves.**

Please remember the above points and add to them any which you may think of yourself. The 10 Dimensions above are not intended to be an authoritative or exhaustive list. They are there to support the "water based analogy" which has worked wel for me and most of the other people I know or have heard from. See if they can help you too.

Appendix 4 – What helps you?

Things that can help <u>YOU</u>.

As a practical way to help you (the sufferer) and their family friends in the future it is important that you always think about ways that improve the way you feel in each of the different feelings when you are feeling depressed. You may not have the same Dimensions (feelings) as others and may have found different feelings which better fit how you feel when you are depressed.

To help you I have attached the following forms which might help you or the family and friends who support you. Every time you remember something that helps (or perhaps more importantly something that makes you feel worse) then you need to write it down.

So why not record it here on the following pages so you know where to find them. I have numbered each of the 10 Dimensions and left them blank so that you can either put in your own Dimensions (feelings) or you can use mine.

I've been asked many times why I don't put in some examples of what can help in each of the following "blank" forms. My answer is always very clear.

We are all different and will be affected differently by the things we choose to do. If I give examples for you to use which don't work for you then you will probably feel inclined to give up trying to find the things which **DO** work. And that will **NOT** be of help to you which is the last thing I want to happen.

You need to choose the things that **DO** work for **YOU** (and perhaps those closest to you) and only **YOU** can do this. You can't get anyone else to do this for you. Whatever time it takes you to work out what works for **YOU** will be time well spent.

Dimension 1	Sea Wave
Relates to the Feeling	Overall feeling of Depression
Your feeling if different	

Things that help this Dimension (feeling) get better for you.

Things that make this Dimension (feeling) worse for you.

Dimension 2	River Current
Relates to the Feeling	Anxiety and Panic Attacks
Your feeling if different	

Things that help this Dimension (feeling) get better for you.

Things that make this Dimension (feeling) worse for you.

Dimension 3	Lake Shore
Relates to the Feeling	Isolation and Vulnerability
Your feeling if different	

Things that help this Dimension (feeling) get better for you.

Things that make this Dimension (feeling) worse for you.

Dimension 4	Time
Relates to the Feeling	Need for and benefit from Support
Your feeling if different	

Things that help this Dimension (feeling) get better for you.

Things that make this Dimension (feeling) worse for you.

Dimension 5	Temperature
Relates to the Feeling	Despair
Your feeling if different	

Things that help this Dimension (feeling) get better for you.

Things that make this Dimension (feeling) worse for you.

Dimension 6	Pressure
Relates to the Feeling	Motivation
Your feeling if different	

Things that help this Dimension (feeling) get better for you.

Things that make this Dimension (feeling) worse for you.

Dimension 7	Wind
Relates to the Feeling	Confidence
Your feeling if different	

Things that help this Dimension (feeling) get better for you.

Things that make this Dimension (feeling) worse for you.

Dimension 8	Rain
Relates to the Feeling	Stress
Your feeling if different	

Things that help this Dimension (feeling) get better for you.

Things that make this Dimension (feeling) worse for you.

Dimension 9	Stars
Relates to the Feeling	Confusion and Memory Loss
Your feeling if different	

Things that help this Dimension (feeling) get better for you.

Things that make this Dimension (feeling) worse for you.

Dimension 10	Sun
Relates to the Feeling	Hope
Your feeling if different	

Things that help this Dimension (feeling) get better for you.

Things that make this Dimension (feeling) worse for you.